PSYCHOLOGICAL ASSESSMENT OF ADULT POSTTRAUMATIC STATES

Erin M. Eadie and John Briere have masterfully summarized the research and provided essential knowledge about psychological trauma and the assessment of its effects. This landmark book guides readers about assessing reactions to trauma ranging from one-time events to complex, developmental traumas, neglect, and social maltreatment. It is a must-have reference for all clinicians.

—**Bethany L. Brand, PhD,** Professor Emerit of Psychology, Towson University, Towson, MD, United States; author of *The Concise Guide to the Assessment and Treatment of Trauma-Related Dissociation,* and coauthor of *Finding Solid Ground: Overcoming Obstacles in Trauma Treatment* and *The Finding Solid Ground Program Workbook: Overcoming Obstacles in Trauma Recovery*

To call this book brilliant and revolutionary is an understatement. The authors are willing to state, clearly and unequivocally, that the domain of trauma includes many things not previously considered and that are not yet included in formal diagnostic manuals. It is solidly based in empirical data, and extremely useful for anyone assessing the effects of the widest possible range of traumas. The authors bring their authority to what is, in effect, a decolonizing of trauma assessment. I am so grateful for this work.

—**Laura S. Brown, PhD, ABPP,** Courtesy Clinical Professor, Department of Psychiatry and Behavioral Sciences, University of Washington, Seattle, United States; author of *Decolonizing Trauma Healing: Toward a Humble, Culturally Responsive Practice*

Eadie and Briere offer a thorough exploration of the intricate phenomenology of posttraumatic stress, and present a cutting-edge approach to the nuanced assessment of trauma-related symptoms. This is an essential read for clinicians working with individuals affected by trauma.

—**Ruth A. Lanius, MD, PhD,** Professor of Psychiatry, Harris-Woodman Chair, University of Western Ontario, London, ON, Canada

Since the publication of the first edition of *Psychological Assessment of Adult Posttraumatic States*, our understanding of the range and scope of traumatic stressors has expanded considerably. In this revised edition, Eadie and Briere provide a review of contemporary viewpoints regarding traumatic stressors and discuss their etiology and range of possible posttraumatic and other consequences, including the complications posed by repeated and cumulative forms of different types of trauma and those based on developmental and diversity issues. On this foundation, they then provide up-to-date information on the use of various instruments, interviews, and strategies—including telehealth methodologies—for assessing traumatized individuals. A very timely resource for those seeking approaches and methods for understanding and documenting a wide variety of posttraumatic consequences.

—**Christine A. Courtois, PhD, ABPP,** Delaware Licensed Psychologist, Board Certified Counseling Psychologist; author of *Healing the Incest Wound: Adult Survivors in Therapy;* coeditor of *Treating Complex Traumatic Stress Disorders in Adults* and coauthor of *Treatment of Complex Trauma: A Sequenced, Relationship-Based Approach*

This text offers an exceedingly rare combination of (a) deep clinical knowledge and extraordinary clinical sensitivity, (b) respect for and knowledge of the trauma literature, (c) solid methodology and statistical skill, and (d) compelling and readable prose. It would be hard to find a better resource for the trauma professional at any level of training. This is one of the very few books that should be both a requirement in a trauma psychology course and a staple in the library of any trauma-informed professional.

—**Constance Dalenberg, PhD,** Distinguished Professor, Alliant International University; Director, Trauma Research Institute, Claremont, CA, United States; Science Committee Chair, Division 56 (Trauma Psychology), American Psychological Association

PSYCHOLOGICAL ASSESSMENT OF ADULT POSTTRAUMATIC STATES

Phenomenology, Diagnosis, and Measurement

Third Edition

Erin M. Eadie and John Briere

 AMERICAN PSYCHOLOGICAL ASSOCIATION

Published by
American Psychological Association
750 First Street, NE
Washington, DC 20002
https://www.apa.org

Order Department
https://www.apa.org/pubs/books
order@apa.org

Typeset in Charter and Interstate by Circle Graphics, Inc., Reisterstown, MD

Printer: Gasch Printing, Odenton, MD
Cover Designer: Gwen J. Grafft, Minneapolis, MN

Library of Congress Cataloging-in-Publication Data

Names: Briere, John, author. | Eadie, Erin, author.
Title: Psychological assessment of adult posttraumatic states :
    phenomenology, diagnosis, and measurement / by Erin Eadie and John
    Briere.
Description: Third edition. | Washington, DC : American Psychological
    Association, [2025] | John Briere's name appears first in the previous
    edition. | Includes bibliographical references and index.
Identifiers: LCCN 2024045853 (print) | LCCN 2024045854 (ebook) | ISBN
    9781433836374 (paperback) | ISBN 9781433841071 (ebook)
Subjects: MESH: Stress Disorders, Post-Traumatic--diagnosis | Adult
Classification: LCC RC552.P67 (print) | LCC RC552.P67 (ebook) | NLM WM
    172.5 | DDC 616.85/21--dc23/eng/20250111
LC record available at https://lccn.loc.gov/2024045853
LC ebook record available at https://lccn.loc.gov/2024045854

https://doi.org/10.1037/0000452-000

Printed in the United States of America

10 9 8 7 6 5 4 3 2 1

Contents

Preface

Professional awareness of posttraumatic distress and disorder is relatively new when compared with more traditional areas of psychological research and clinical practice. Although there have been anecdotal reports of the psychological effects of wars and natural disasters throughout history, most of the empirically validated information on the impact of interpersonal violence, disasters, and other traumatic events has been published since the early to mid-1980s. As a result, mental health professionals have had access to less clinical information regarding posttraumatic stress than, for example, similar information on anxiety, depression, or psychosis. Fortunately, our knowledge of psychological trauma, as well as the availability of validated trauma-specific assessment devices, has increased dramatically during the past several decades.

Although the first two editions of *Psychological Assessment of Adult Posttraumatic States: Phenomenology, Diagnosis, and Measurement* summarized this emerging literature and reviewed a range of trauma-related tests and interviews, the most recent edition was published in 2004. Since then, our understanding of psychological trauma, its effects, and how to assess them has grown dramatically. At the same time, some early assessment instruments have fallen out of favor because (a) they relate to early, no longer applied diagnostic systems (e.g., the *Diagnostic and Statistical Manual of Mental Disorders, Third Edition* [*DSM-III*], or *Fourth Edition, Text Revision* [*DSM-IV-TR*]; American Psychiatric Association, 1980, 2000); (b) their psychometric characteristics did not meet current standards; or (c) other, more recently developed measures were found to be more useful.

The third edition of *Psychological Assessment of Adult Posttraumatic States* summarizes the most relevant and recent research on posttraumatic disturbance as well as new information on traumas or adversities covered less in previous editions. Here, we discuss complex, cumulative, and developmental traumas; parental disattunement and emotional neglect; drug-facilitated sexual assault; sex trafficking; pregnancy loss; COVID-19–related stressors; and exposure to social maltreatment, such as racism, sexism, transphobia, and microaggressions. We also consider psychological syndromes or disorders that have only recently come to light, such as complex PTSD, disturbed self-capacities and self-organization, prolonged grief disorder, distress reduction behaviors, and somatic and functional neurological symptom disorders. Also included in this regard are those trauma-related disorders whose symptoms or characteristics were substantially updated in the fifth edition of the *DSM* (*DSM-5*) and its text revision (*DSM-5-TR*; American Psychiatric Association, 2013, 2022), such as PTSD, acute stress disorder, the dissociative disorders, the adjustment disorders, and borderline personality disorder.

Most importantly, this edition reviews currently available psychological tests and interviews as they relate to trauma and adversity—both those developed to specifically address posttraumatic effects and those considered more generic that can nevertheless be helpful in evaluating comorbidities and some posttraumatic outcomes. Many previously available generic tests, such as the Minnesota Multiphasic Personality Inventory–2 (MMPI-2; Ben-Porath & Tellegen, 2008), the Personality Assessment Inventory (PAI; Morey, 1991), and the Millon Clinical Multiaxial Inventory–III (MCMI-III; Millon, 1994), have been updated since publication of the second edition of this book. Some trauma-specific measures, such as the Trauma Symptom Inventory (TSI; Briere, 1995) and the Clinician-Administered PTSD Scale (CAPS; Blake et al., 1990, 1995), also have been revised substantially, requiring new descriptions and discussion in this book regarding their clinical utility in modern trauma assessment practice. As well, the COVID-19 pandemic saw the rise of teleassessment approaches involving tablets, computers, and telephones using modern, Health Insurance Portability and Accountability Act–compliant platforms (e.g., Zoom and Webex). Teleassessment approaches are described and reviewed in Chapter 8 (new to this volume).

Although children also experience a variety of difficulties in response to major stressors, this book is limited to adult posttraumatic responses. The interested reader is referred to Denton et al. (2017), Eklund et al. (2018), Friedrich (2002), Kisiel et al. (2021), Nader (2004), Strand et al. (2005), and the National Child Traumatic Stress Network (2024) for information specific to the assessment of traumatized children and adolescents.

Acknowledgments

The authors would like to thank those who provided feedback on the third edition of this book, supported us in its writing, and informed our assessment thinking over the years. These individuals include Judith Armstrong, Bethany Brand, Eve Carlson, Chris Courtois, Constance Dalenberg, Elaine Eaton, Diana Elliott, Amy Escott, Julian Ford, Bill Friedrich, Natacha Godbout, Ruth Lanius, Cheryl Lanktree, Alana Newman, Marsha Runtz, Randye Semple, and Frank Weathers.

Erin is immensely thankful to her family, in particular her husband, parents, in-laws, and especially her two children, who showed incredible patience and provided many creative and indisputable reasons to take (much-needed) breaks during the writing process. She would also like to thank Alia Kuraishi, Jennifer Hilborn, Julie Irwin, Madalyn Marcus, Virginia Schenk, and the many other friends and colleagues who provided thoughtful input, personal experiences, and clinical insights that enriched the contents of this book.

John also thanks Cheryl Lanktree for the many years of love, support, and partnership as well as for her feedback on this book.

Finally, the authors are deeply grateful to the many clients and patients whose lived experiences have informed the development and ongoing evolution of trauma-relevant assessment and trauma-informed care.

PSYCHOLOGICAL ASSESSMENT OF ADULT POSTTRAUMATIC STATES

PART I ETIOLOGY AND PHENOMENOLOGY OF POSTTRAUMATIC STRESS

1 TRAUMA TYPES, CHARACTERISTICS, AND COMPLEXITY

Although the psychological literature indicates that trauma exposure is associated with a wide range of symptoms, problems, and disorders, these effects often vary according to the type of adverse experience as well as its severity, duration, onset, complexity, whether it was interpersonal, and other important characteristics. Furthermore, it turns out that many adverse events that do not meet the *Diagnostic and Statistical Manual of Mental Disorders, Fifth Edition, Text Revision* (*DSM-5-TR*) trauma criteria (American Psychiatric Association, 2022) can lead to posttraumatic symptomatology. In this chapter, we outline the issues associated with defining trauma, explore the various traumas and serious adverse events known to produce posttraumatic symptoms, and consider the various peri- and posttraumatic factors (e.g., immediate emotional and dissociative responses, social support, and responsiveness) that mediate or moderate psychological symptoms.

https://doi.org/10.1037/0000452-001
Psychological Assessment of Adult Posttraumatic States: Phenomenology, Diagnosis, and Measurement, Third Edition, by E. M. Eadie and J. Briere

DEFINING TRAUMA

Unlike most other diagnostic categories in the *DSM-5-TR*, the diagnoses of posttraumatic stress disorder (PTSD) and acute stress disorder (ASD) require a specific evaluation of etiology as well as symptomatology. Because the *DSM-5-TR* diagnostic criteria require the presence of a major stressor (referred to as *Criterion A*) before a diagnosis of PTSD can be made, the clinician must not only assess symptoms of stress but also evaluate the nature of the stressor, including when the stressor is sufficiently severe to warrant the term *trauma*.

Assessment of trauma exposure may appear to be a simple matter of listing those events known to produce posttraumatic stress; however, the wide variety of adverse experiences that might be included defies easy categorization. Furthermore, it is now clear that an event that produces posttraumatic stress in one individual may not do so in another. Perhaps most importantly, it is often not one discrete event that comprises the experience of trauma; in many cases, such as war, torture, or interpersonal violence, a series of linked events encompass the traumatic experience.

A notable change in the *DSM-5-TR* criteria for PTSD (and ASD), compared with previous editions, is the option to include posttraumatic symptoms that arise from, or are related to, different traumatic events (Briere & Scott, 2015). For example, in contrast to previous *DSM* editions, nightmares can now be related to one trauma (e.g., sexual assault) and effortful avoidance to another (e.g., motor vehicle accident) and both symptoms can count toward a diagnosis of PTSD. In the past, all symptoms of PTSD or ASD had to be linked to the same single traumatic event, potentially leading to underdiagnosis of individuals with histories of multiple traumas and symptoms arising from different traumatic events (T. L. Simpson et al., 2011). This change is a marked improvement because it recognizes, as discussed throughout this book, that posttraumatic symptoms often reflect the cumulative experiences of multiple, repeated, and often complex traumatic events.

The *DSM-5-TR* diagnostic criteria for PTSD and ASD define trauma as follows:

- Exposure to actual or threatened death, serious injury, or sexual violence in one (or more) of the following ways:
  - Directly experiencing the traumatic event(s).
  - Witnessing, in person (not through the media), the event(s) as it occurred to others.
  - Learning that the traumatic event(s) occurred to a close family member or close friend—in cases of actual or threatened death of a family member or friend, the event(s) must have been violent or accidental.

- Experiencing repeated or extreme exposure to aversive details of the traumatic event(s) during work (e.g., first responders collecting human remains; police officers repeatedly exposed to details of child abuse). Of note, this does not apply to exposure through electronic media, television, movies, or pictures, unless this exposure is occupationally related. (American Psychiatric Association, 2022, pp. 301, 313–314)

A notable improvement in the *DSM-5-TR* is the expansion of the fourth edition definition (*DSM-IV*; American Psychiatric Association, 1994) of what constitutes sexual violence. The *DSM-5-TR* definition now includes the following:

> forced sexual penetration; alcohol/drug-facilitated nonconsensual sexual penetration; other unwanted sexual contact; and other unwanted sexual experiences not involving contact, such as being forced to watch pornography, exposure to the display of genitals by an exhibitionist, or being the victim of unwanted photography or videotaping of a sexual nature or the unwanted dissemination of these photographs or videos. (American Psychiatric Association, 2022, p. 305)

This expanded definition is consistent with the previous specification in the *DSM-IV* that in childhood, "sexually traumatic events may include developmentally inappropriate sexual experiences *without threatened or actual violence or injury*" (American Psychiatric Association, 2000, p. 464, emphasis added). Although there is some debate about what experiences should be considered abusive sexual contact or noncontact sexual abuse (e.g., Levin et al., 2014), the broadening of this criterion allows inclusion of victimization experiences that previously might not have been technically considered a trauma (e.g., drug-facilitated sexual contact with someone who could not render consent, or some cases of sexual harassment) but that can nevertheless result in posttraumatic stress or other adverse outcomes (Avina & O'Donohue, 2002; Gauntlett-Gilbert et al., 2004).

Using this or similar (i.e., *DSM-IV*) definitions, it is estimated that approximately 80% of adults in the United States have undergone, or will undergo, at least one major trauma in their lifetime (e.g., Benjet et al., 2016; Kilpatrick et al., 2013). Yet, as we will see, if threats not involving potential death or injury were included in the *DSM-5-TR* (or the prior edition), this percentage would be even higher. Prevalence data of this magnitude highlight the ubiquity of trauma exposure in North America—not just in clinical settings but in the general population as well.

Beyond Criterion A

Even with improvements made to *DSM-5-TR* Criterion A for PTSD and ASD, there are significant criticisms. Perhaps most importantly, the requirement that a trauma involve "exposure to actual or threatened death, serious injury, or sexual violence" (American Psychiatric Association, 2022, p. 301) is potentially problematic because many events seemingly can be traumatic even if life threat, injury, or violence is not present (Anders et al. 2011; Briere & Scott, 2014). In contrast, the revised third edition (*DSM-III-R*; American Psychiatric Association, 1987) included threats to psychological integrity (e.g., extreme emotional abuse, nonviolent loss of a loved one, or extended humiliation or degradation) as long as they were "outside the range of usual human experience and that would be markedly distressing to almost anyone" (p. 250). Threats to psychological integrity were removed in the *DSM-IV* definition and are not present in the *DSM-5* or *DSM-5-TR*. Yet by excluding events if they are highly upsetting but not life-threatening, the *DSM-5-TR* diagnostic criteria may underestimate the extent of actual trauma in the general population and reduce the availability of a stress disorder diagnosis for some individuals who would otherwise meet all other criteria for ASD or PTSD.

Given the potential limitations of *DSM-5-TR* Criterion A, some have suggested that the term *trauma* be broadened as it applies to modern clinical practice. When considering the broader effects of trauma and when assessing for the purposes of treatment planning, it may be helpful to consider a more inclusive definition. For example, Briere and Scott (2014) suggested that "[A]n event is traumatic if it is extremely upsetting, at least temporarily overwhelms the individual's internal resources, and produces lasting psychological distress" (p. 4). This broader definition includes experiences such as sudden, severe emotional losses (see Carlson et al., 2013), extreme parental neglect or abandonment (Sroufe et al., 2005), and moral injury (Shay, 2014) and thus addresses the concerns of people who might benefit from trauma-informed therapies. It also reflects the fact that people who experience major challenges to psychological integrity can suffer as much as those traumatized by physical injury or immediate life threat. This is primarily a treatment issue, however; for the purpose of formally diagnosing a stress disorder, clinicians should adhere to the *DSM-5-TR* definition of trauma.

Complex and Cumulative Trauma

As noted earlier, the *DSM-5* (American Psychiatric Association, 2013) abandoned the single trauma requirement of previous *DSM* editions (Briere & Scott, 2015) and now specifies symptom criteria that arise from traumatic "event(s)." This transition from a single event to a potentially multitrauma criterion highlights a theme that we will return to throughout this book: Significant trauma-related symptoms are often the result of multiple additive or interactive stressors that accumulate and potentially operate synergistically over time (Briere, Runtz, et al., 2020; Briggs et al., 2021). This change is especially relevant to some more commonly occurring traumas that tend to involve multiple events, contexts, and interactions, not all of which conform to *DSM-5-TR* Criterion A. These include not only severe interpersonal abuse, harassment, and related experiences but also social discrimination and maltreatment of marginalized groups and individuals, arising from systemic racism, sexism, transphobia, and xenophobia (Briere et al., 2025; S. T. Russell & Fish, 2016; Sue et al., 2007; M. T. Williams, 2021).

As described later in this chapter, abuse and other childhood adversities may produce symptoms and maladaptive behaviors in adolescence and adulthood that increase the likelihood of later victimization. These later traumas may then lead to further behaviors and responses (e.g., substance abuse, gang activities) that are additional risk factors for further trauma exposure and potentially even more complex mental health outcomes. The accumulation of multiple, different forms of interpersonal trauma over the lifespan is sometimes referred to as *cumulative trauma* (e.g., Briere et al., 2008; Cloitre et al., 2009; Follette et al., 1996) and, when it results in multiple psychological symptoms and problems, *complex trauma* (Courtois, 2004; J. L. Herman, 1992a). Although cumulative childhood traumas appear to be, on average, more impactful than adult ones (Cloitre et al., 2009), multiple experiences of highly aversive adult traumas (e.g., torture, sustained relational violence, prisoner-of-war experiences) can also result in complex posttraumatic outcomes (e.g., J. L. Herman, 1992b). Studies indicate that cumulative interpersonal traumas are more likely than single ones to lead to a diagnosis of PTSD or ASD (Briere, Agee, & Dietrich, 2016; Briere, Dias, et al., 2017; Karam et al., 2014) and to produce more complex symptomatology (Briere et al., 2008; Cloitre et al., 2009; Felitti & Anda, 2003).

The fact that childhood and adult adversities and traumas can accumulate to produce a range of psychological difficulties has implications for the assessment of both trauma exposure and trauma outcomes. For example, current symptoms in an adult trauma survivor might represent the following:

- the lasting effects of childhood abuse and/or neglect, social maltreatment, and insecure attachment that have persisted into adulthood;

- the effects of more recent sexual or physical assaults, emotional abuse, social maltreatment, or other traumas;

- the additive/cumulative effects of childhood and adult traumas and adversities; and/or

- the exacerbation of earlier, childhood traumas as a function of more recent adult adversities.

In the latter instance, especially severe, regressed, dissociated, or self-destructive responses to an adult trauma may arise, in part, from its interaction with early adversities and trauma, such as when traumatic childhood memories are triggered by more recent mistreatment or trauma, resulting in more severe or complex symptom presentations.

The mixture of multiple traumas, multiple risks, endemic social maltreatment, and multiple symptomatic responses is well known to trauma-focused clinicians, who sometimes find it difficult (a) to connect certain symptoms to certain traumas and other symptoms to other traumas or (b) to discriminate trauma-related symptoms from less trauma-specific ones. The remaining chapters of this book describe assessment approaches that clarify these various trauma–symptom connections and, in some cases, provide alternative ways of conceptualizing complex trauma and multisymptom presentations.

SPECIFIC STRESSORS KNOWN TO PRODUCE POSTTRAUMATIC SYMPTOMS

Although there are many potentially traumatic events, a smaller subset of these is cited regularly in the literature as producing posttraumatic symptomatology. Several of these more common stressors are described briefly in terms of their incidence and potential posttraumatic effects. It is important to reiterate that these (and other) traumatic events are often well within the range of normal human experience. In fact, surveys suggest that up to 80% of people in the general population have experienced at least one major traumatic stressor (Benjet et al., 2016; Norris, 1992; Resnick et al., 1993). If major threats to psychological integrity are also counted, this proportion would be even higher. Although such traumatic stressors are common, their ability to produce significant posttraumatic disturbance varies as a function of a wide variety of other variables, as discussed in Chapter 2 (this volume).

Interpersonal Versus Noninterpersonal Traumas

One of the most significant of these variables is whether the event was due to nonhuman factors (e.g., earthquakes, floods, or tornadoes), resulted from unintended acts (e.g., motor vehicle accidents), or arose from intended interpersonal violence (e.g., rape or physical assault). In general, assault or abuse by another person is associated with substantially more posttraumatic disturbance than are natural disasters or unintended acts. In a study directly comparing the effects of disasters to interpersonal violence in the general population, Briere and Elliott (2000) found that interpersonal victimization was associated with far greater symptomatology than was disaster exposure. The same study indicated, however, that disasters also were quite capable of producing negative, albeit less common, mental health outcomes that persisted for many years.

Developmental Trauma

Research over the last several decades indicates that although traumas experienced in adulthood can have major psychological effects, childhood traumas may be even more detrimental (Teicher et al., 2022). Such developmental traumas, which include the various forms of maltreatment outlined in this chapter, occur during the most vulnerable points in human development and tend to continue over long periods of time (Cook et al., 2005; Courtois, 2004). Developmental trauma can result not only in the posttraumatic symptoms sometimes found in survivors of adult traumas but also in altered self-capacities and disrupted parent–child attachment, including problems with emotional regulation, identity, and formation of stable interpersonal relationships (Bachem et al., 2021; Bigras et al., 2015; Briere & Rickards, 2007). Unfortunately, research indicates that early abuse and neglect may be associated with poorer response to both psychotherapy and psychiatric medication relative to adult-onset traumas (e.g., Nemeroff et al., 2003). Although most types of traumas can occur at any point in the human lifespan (e.g., a hurricane, a house fire, or a motor vehicle accident), these are typically not considered to be developmental traumas because they do not exclusively occur in childhood and do not inherently disrupt caregiver–child attachment relationships.

Sexual and Physical Abuse

Childhood sexual and physical maltreatment are quite prevalent in North American society. Retrospective self-report studies suggest that more than 20% of women and 5% of men in the United States describe being sexually abused as children or adolescents (e.g., Finkelhor et al., 2014). Briere, Runtz, and colleagues (2020) found that 36% of individuals in an online sample of North American women had experienced unwanted sexual contact at age 13 years or younger. When sexual abuse is defined as including non-contact victimization (e.g., sexual comments, propositions) during childhood or adolescence, the prevalence is roughly double that of contact sexual abuse alone (Briere et al., 2024). Several meta-analyses indicate that childhood sexual abuse can be broadly impactful; it is associated with a variety of psychological and social symptoms and disorders (e.g., Hailes et al., 2019; Paolucci et al., 2001).

Similarly, between 10% and 22% of men and women report experiences of physical abuse in childhood (e.g., Briere & Elliott, 2003), minimally defined as caregiver behavior that resulted in injuries such as cuts, bruises, or broken bones. It should be noted, however, that retrospective self-reports of childhood trauma vary according to study, research methodology, geography, and participant willingness to disclose (Stoltenborgh et al., 2011), making it difficult to assess the exact prevalence of child maltreatment in North America or elsewhere.

Psychological Maltreatment

Psychological abuse, characterized by caregiver behaviors that involve excessive and continuing criticism, denigration, blaming, insults, and threats (e.g., Hart et al., 2011), is common in the general population. Rates vary widely depending on how inclusive a definition is used. For example, almost all individuals will endorse at least one item on a continuous measure of psychological abuse in childhood (e.g., "Did your parents criticize you?") because these experiences are relatively common at low frequencies (Briere et al., 2012; Straus et al., 1998; Van Bruggen et al., 2006; D. A. Wolfe & McIsaac, 2011). However, assessments of repeated and persistent experiences of psychological or emotional abuse in childhood tend to yield estimates of 12% to 22% (e.g., Edwards et al., 2003; Finzi-Dottan & Karu, 2006). Psychological abuse is not always considered as serious as sexual or physical maltreatment, and because these experiences do not always involve immediate threats to life or physical integrity, they rarely meet *DSM-5-TR* trauma criteria. This assumption can be incorrect, however: Chronic psychological abuse is a major life stressor with a range of long-term psychological effects (Briere et al., 2012; Teicher et al., 2006; Yun et al., 2019). In some cases, psychological maltreatment is an even stronger predictor of adverse outcomes than other forms of maltreatment (e.g., Spinazzola et al., 2014).

Psychological Neglect, Disattunement, and Insecure Attachment

Although it is not included in *DSM-5-TR* Criterion A, early psychological neglect and disattunement can be powerfully adverse experiences that play a significant role in the psychosocial difficulties of many (Sroufe et al., 2005). *Psychological neglect* generally involves inadequate parental attention, protection, nurturance, and affection, whereas *disattunement* refers to disengaged parental caretaking, such as ignoring or not noticing the child's needs, nonresponsiveness to the child's proximity-seeking behavior, or, in some cases, dissociation or substance abuse that interferes with normal parental responsivity (Briere, Runtz, et al., 2017). Early neglect and disattunement can be potent sources of psychosocial difficulties involving disturbances in self-organization (DSOs; Bachem et al., 2021)—primarily, difficulties with self-concept, relational functioning, and emotional regulation (Ford & Courtois, 2021; Levy et al., 2015)—as discussed in Chapter 2.

The relationship between childhood neglect or disattunement (as well as other forms of early maltreatment) and DSOs highlights the foundational nature of parent–child attachment. Early parent–child interactions that are characterized by neglect, disattunement, rejection, or significant loss often lead to insecure attachment (J. A. Simpson & Rholes, 2015). For this reason, modern theorists tend to view caregiver disattunement and neglect as potentially quite traumatic and harmful, even though they generally do not meet *DSM-5-TR* criteria for a traumatic event.

Witnessing Intimate Partner Violence

An additional form of psychological and health-related harm during childhood is witnessing household violence, particularly between parental figures (Forke et al., 2019; D. A. Wolfe et al., 2003). In the often-cited studies of adverse childhood experiences (ACEs), Felitti and colleagues (1998) found that approximately 12% of adults recalled being exposed to violence toward their mother or stepmother during their childhood. Long-term effects of witnessing intimate partner violence (IPV) include alcoholism, illicit drug use, and depression (Dube et al., 2002) as well as a variety of other symptoms and problems (Holt et al., 2008).

Child Maltreatment–Related Revictimization

Child maltreatment not only can produce enduring psychological dysfunction, it is also associated with a greater likelihood of being sexually or physically revictimized later in life (Duckworth & Follette, 2011). This association may be largest for childhood sexual abuse and later sexual assault (e.g., Van Bruggen et al., 2006). In one study, women who reported experiencing sexual abuse in childhood had twice the likelihood of later sexual assault (68%) than those without a history of sexual abuse (34%; Briere, Runtz, et al., 2020). In that research, child abuse not only increased the likelihood of later trauma, but both childhood and adult traumas also additively contributed to elevated levels of psychological distress and dysfunction.

Adult Rape and Sexual Assault

Rape can be defined as nonconsensual oral, anal, or vaginal sexual penetration of an adolescent or adult with a body part or object, through the use of threat or physical force, or when the victim is incapable of giving consent. The term *sexual assault* sometimes refers to any forced sexual contact short of rape, although we will define it more broadly in this book as any forced sexual contact, including rape.

The prevalence of sexual assault among adult women in the United States is reported to be between 15% and 22% (Black et al., 2011; Elliott et al., 2004; Tjaden & Thoennes, 2000). This statistic may be an underestimation for some groups, however. For example, research with university women often reveals higher rates (Eadie et al., 2008; Tansill et al., 2012), with one study finding that 19% of university women reported attempted or completed sexual assault since entering college alone (Krebs et al., 2009). When adolescent girls are included, the prevalence of sexual assault is generally higher. In one study, 32% of women had experienced unwanted sexual contact at age 14 or later (Briere, Runtz, et al., 2020). Sexual assault rates for men are less clear but are estimated to range between 2% and 5% (Black et al., 2011; Elliott et al., 2004).

Drug-Facilitated Sexual Assault

Drug-facilitated sexual assault (DFSA) involves the use of drugs or alcohol to incapacitate potential victims, who can then be sexually assaulted without resistance (Butler & Welch, 2009). The most frequently used substances in DFSA are alcohol, benzodiazepines, antihistamines, antidepressants, muscle relaxants, scopolamine, GHB (γ-hydroxybutyrate), and ketamine (Fiorentin & Logan, 2019). In some cases, perpetrators victimize already intoxicated people or coerce future victims into overusing alcohol or drugs. In others, the drug is administered covertly, such as in an unguarded drink at a bar.

Military Sexual Trauma

Clinicians and researchers have increasingly documented the phenomenon of military sexual trauma, involving sexual coercion and assaults against active-duty personnel by their peers or command superiors in the military (e.g., Ormerod & Steel, 2018). In a meta-analysis of 69 studies, L. C. Wilson (2018) found that 24% of female military personnel and veterans reported instances of sexual assault in the military and 53% reported sexual harassment.

Sexual Assault During War or Immigration

A significant number of women and children living in war-torn countries have experienced sexual assault, partially because sexual violence may be used by invading forces as a way to assert control, humiliate civilians, devastate morale, foster "ethnic cleansing" through impregnation, or "reward" soldiers (e.g., Berman et al., 2006; Sawyer, 2009). Women and children are also sometimes sexually assaulted during immigration—for example, by traffickers who sexually assault people as they transport them across the Mexico–U.S. border (Fernandez, 2019).

Physical Assault

Physical assault refers to physical bullying, muggings, beatings, stabbings, shootings, attempted strangulations, and other violent actions against either someone who is known to the assailant or a stranger. Such assaults include violent acts against members of racial and ethnic minority groups and people identifying (or identified) as LGBTQ+, gang-related aggression, work-place violence, and peer assaults. When physical assaults occur within an intimate relationship, they are typically characterized as IPV (discussed next). Although many acts of violence in relationships are directed toward women rather than men, the reverse appears true for physical assaults by strangers (e.g., Currier & Briere, 2000). The U.S. Department of Justice estimated that stranger assaults accounted for approximately 38% of all incidents of nonfatal violence in the United States in 2010 (Harrell, 2012).

Intimate Partner Violence

IPV is usually defined as physically or sexually assaultive behavior by one person against another in an intimate and often cohabiting relationship. Although IPV is usually viewed as victimization of heterosexual women by heterosexual men, there are a number of studies documenting IPV within LGBTQ+ relationships as well as violence against heterosexual men by their partners (Decker et al., 2018; Godbout, Vaillancourt-Morel, et al., 2019). In many cases, there is also emotional abuse, including humiliation, degrada-tion, extreme criticism, and coercive control involving dominance through intimidation, isolation, stalking, and terror-inducting violence or threats of violence (Black et al., 2011; Dichter et al., 2018; Kendall-Tackett, 2009). The U.S. Centers for Disease Control and Prevention National Intimate Partner and Sexual Violence Survey indicated that more than 23% of women and 13% of men have experienced severe physical violence by an intimate partner at some point in their lives, whereas 16% of women and 7% of men have experienced contact sexual violence from a partner (S. G. Smith et al., 2017).

Commercial Sexual Exploitation

Sexual exploitation for commercial purposes is similar in many ways to child-hood and adult sexual assault, but with the abuser or trafficker benefitting financially or in some other commercial way. Often these traumas are multiple and layered, involving extensive coercive control, force, or both, with the exploited individual treated as a commodity.

Sex Trafficking

Sex trafficking can be defined as the forced or coerced recruitment, transportation, transfer, harboring, or receipt of individuals, both children and adults, for the purposes of commercial sexual exploitation (The Protection Project, 2011). It is estimated that 15,000 to 18,000 people are trafficked into the United States each year for sex or forced labor (U.S. Department of State, 2005), whereupon they may be forced into prostitution, pornography, or work in massage parlors or for escort services (e.g., Ugarte et al., 2004).

Prostitution

Research indicates that most people engaged in prostitution are marginalized by race, poverty, gender identity, and low education (e.g., Monroe, 2005); frequently have histories of childhood trauma (e.g., McClanahan et al., 1999); and are more likely to be addicted to drugs (e.g., Young et al., 2000). In addition, a significant proportion are minors (Institute of Medicine & National Research Council, 2013). Studies suggest that those involved in prostitution have at least a 40% to 80% probability of being raped (Farley & Barkan, 1998; Valera et al., 2000) and undergo considerable physical and emotional abuse (Farley, 2017; Miller & Schwartz, 1995; Vanwesenbeeck et al., 1995). Prostitution is often injurious to physical and psychological health and is a substantial risk factor for homicide and serious injury (e.g., Farley, 2004b). Notably, some people eschew the label *prostitution*, instead using the less stigmatizing term *sex work* (K. J. Bell, 2009; Open Society, 2019). It should be noted, however, that when such activity occurs when the person is a minor or is under the control of another person or when sex acts occur in the context of nonconsent, force, or coercion, the term may be misleading because it falsely implies a freely chosen behavior or occupation (Moran & Farley, 2018). In instances involving minors, the term *commercial sexual exploitation of children* is more appropriate.

Torture

Torture can be defined as follows:

> any act by which severe pain or suffering, whether physical or mental, is intentionally inflicted on a person for such purposes as obtaining from him [*sic*] or a third person information or confession, punishing him for an act he has committed or is suspected of having committed, or intimidating him or a third person. (United Nations Treaty Collection, 1984)

Amnesty International (2015) reported that 141 nations sanction or tacitly allow the use of torture, and a meta-analysis suggested that more than 1 million torture-surviving refugees currently reside in the United States (Higson-Smith, 2015). Torture survivors are especially overrepresented among refugees, with the Center for Victims of Torture estimating that 44% of refugees in the United States are either torture survivors or family members or close intimates of survivors (Higson-Smith, 2015).

Mass Casualty Events

Large-scale events that cause widespread fear, terror, injury, and physical casualties can have significant psychological effects on many individuals in a specific venue, community, or geographic area. These events can be interpersonal in nature, as is the case with a terrorist attack or a mass shooting, or noninterpersonal in origin, such as a natural disaster or transportation accident.

Interpersonal Violence

Violence committed outside of war by one or more people and involving high numbers of injuries or casualties has existed throughout human history. Recent examples in the United States include the Oklahoma City bombing of 1995, the 9/11 attacks on the World Trade Center and the Pentagon in 2001, the Sandy Hook school shooting in 2012, the Las Vegas mass shooting in 2017, and the school shooting in Parkland, Florida, in 2018.

Natural Disasters

Natural disasters can be defined as large-scale, not directly human-caused, injury- or death-producing environmental events that adversely affect a significant number of people. They are relatively common in the United States, with 13% to 30% of individuals having experienced one or more natural disasters in their lifetime (Briere & Elliott, 2000; Green & Solomon, 1995). Typical disasters include earthquakes, large fires, floods, tsunamis, avalanches, hurricanes, and tornadoes.

Large-Scale Transportation Accidents

Transportation accidents include airplane crashes, train derailments, and maritime accidents that often involve multiple victims and high fatality rates (Maeda & Higa, 2006). Large-scale accidents can be especially traumatic to survivors because they frequently occur over a relatively extended period of time, during which the victims are exposed to ongoing terror and fear of death.

Fire and Burns

Beyond fire-related disasters, a significant number of survivors seen by trauma clinicians have experienced injury by smaller fires. These include house fires, often caused by smoking in bed, electrical short circuits, or leaking or malfunctioning propane tanks, stoves, or heaters, as well as fires that occur in recreational contexts, involving barbecues, firepits, and fireworks. Serious burns also may result from motor vehicle accidents, industrial fires, or even intentional attacks by others. In the United States alone, more than 32,000 people are hospitalized for severe burns each year (American Burn Association, 2024). The potential physical effects of serious burns—including extreme pain, a long recovery period, multiple surgeries, visible or painful scars (or both), disfigurement, amputation, and reduced mobility—mean that burn trauma can continue and repeat over time (Gilboa et al., 1994; L. Martin et al., 2017).

Motor Vehicle Accidents

It is estimated that approximately 20% of individuals in the United States have experienced a serious motor vehicle accident (Blanchard & Hickling, 2004). A substantial number develop psychological symptoms (e.g., A. Craig et al., 2016), especially if the accident involved major injuries or resulted in the death of others (Blanchard et al., 2003). When the driver is responsible for the accident, guilt and self-blame may increase subsequent psychological symptoms (Fitzharris et al., 2005). Survivors of a major motor vehicle accident may sustain traumatic brain injury, which can further complicate assessment and treatment (Harvey & Bryant, 2002).

War

War can involve a wide range of violent and traumatic experiences, including immediate threat of death, grievous physical injury, witnessing injury or death (or both) of others, and involvement in injuring or killing people (e.g., Gahm et al., 2007). For those captured, war sometimes includes extended confinement, torture, rape, and extreme physical deprivation. These traumas, in turn, can produce a variety of symptoms and disorders, perhaps especially PTSD (Institute of Medicine, 2010). Although the U.S. Department of Veterans Affairs (VA) provides care for many U.S. war veterans with service-connected injuries, others may not qualify for (or desire) such treatment, and it is not uncommon for veterans to present to non-VA mental health centers and clinicians. For this reason, we recommend (a) that all adult clients be queried regarding any military service and participation in war, and (b) that clinicians be prepared to address war-related trauma in addition to the effects of other adversities. Because the assessment and treatment of combat veterans and others exposed to war can be complex, we recommend clinicians refer to specialized information (e.g., Committee on the Assessment of Ongoing Efforts in the Treatment of Posttraumatic Stress Disorder, Board on the Health of Select Populations, & Institute of Medicine, 2014; B. A. Moore & Penk, 2019) in this area.

War also can profoundly affect the people indigenous to where it takes place, whether through direct military action against noncombatants, forced migration, or degraded social support systems. Living in a war-torn area or armed-conflict zone is associated with significant and lasting anxiety, depression, PTSD, and other adverse outcomes for both children and noncombatant adults (El Baba & Colucci, 2018; Eytan et al., 2011).

Moral Injury

First described by Shay (1995), moral injury involves "perpetrating, failing to prevent, bearing witness to, or learning about acts that transgress deeply held moral beliefs and expectations" (Litz et al., 2009, p. 697). In addition to the grotesqueries of war, command malpractice, and betrayal by cocombatants, recent formulations of war-related moral injury include the act of torturing or killing others, committing or failing to prevent atrocities, using disproportionate violence, giving or following immoral orders, and engaging in violent crimes or accidentally deadly acts against civilians (e.g., Callaway & Spates, 2016).

Of late, the term *moral injury* also has been applied to the experiences of health care professionals, first responders, and others who have engaged in or observed immoral or unfair acts, inadequate care, and difficult ethical dilemmas (Koenig & Al Zaben, 2021). In a recent example, health care workers working with critically ill patients with coronavirus disease 2019 (COVID-19) may report moral injury associated with difficult triage decisions or relative helplessness to adequately treat dying individuals (D'Alessandro et al., 2022). Whatever its source, moral injury can lead to alienation from others or society, lack of trust, loss of meaning, shame, and disruption of religious or spiritual beliefs (Drescher et al., 2011; Koenig et al., 2018), along with more classically clinical outcomes such as anxiety, depression, guilt and self-blame, anger, suicidality, and substance abuse (e.g., Litz et al., 2018).

Traumatic Loss

Traumatic loss generally refers to exposure to the sudden, unexpected death of a loved one or close friend. This may involve witnessing a violent death at the hands of family members, gangs, or police officers, or sudden loss of life associated with mass casualty events, major accidents, and medical events such as a fatal heart attack or sudden death by suicide or disease. Such events may lead to traumatic bereavement, involving extended grief, guilt, anxiety, depression, anger, suicidality, and posttraumatic stress (Boelen et al., 2019; Green et al., 2001; Prigerson et al., 1997). Extended responses to traumatic loss are described in Chapter 2 as part of the new *DSM-5-TR* diagnosis, prolonged grief disorder.

Elder Abuse

Elder abuse includes physical, emotional, or sexual abuse; and/or neglect, abandonment, or financial exploitation of an older person by a caregiver, family member, or other person in a position of trust (American Psychological Association, 2020b; J. E. Hall et al., 2016). It is estimated to affect 1 in 10 people aged 60 years or older in the United States (Acierno et al., 2010; Laumann et al., 2008; National Center on Elder Abuse, 2005). Although all forms of elder abuse can be psychologically devastating (Dong et al., 2013), clinical experience suggests that physical and sexual elder abuse are especially likely to result in classical symptoms of posttraumatic stress.

Stalking

Stalking involves repeatedly following or harassing another person in such a way that they feel terrorized, intimidated, or threatened. In one large study, 8% of women and 2% of men in the United States reported having been stalked by someone; 81% of women who were stalked by a former intimate partner were physically assaulted, and 31% were sexually assaulted (Tjaden & Thoennes, 1998). Although sometimes discounted in U.S. society, especially when no physical violence has transpired, stalking can be traumatizing and result in significant psychological symptomatology, including posttraumatic stress, anxiety, depression, and somatization (Amar, 2006; Hauch & Elklit, 2023).

Life-Threatening Medical Conditions

As opposed to the *DSM-IV*, the *DSM-5* no longer considers many illnesses or medical issues, such as cancer or heart attack, inevitably to be Criterion A–level traumas. It notes that "a life-threatening illness or debilitating medical condition is not necessarily considered a traumatic event. Medical incidents that qualify as traumatic events involve sudden, catastrophic events"

(American Psychiatric Association, 2013, p. 274). As a result, very upsetting medical experiences that might previously have been considered traumatic (e.g., a cancer diagnosis, heart attack, or HIV/AIDS) as well as medical procedures (e.g., heart surgery, invasive cancer treatment, and debridement for severe burns) are not necessarily considered traumatic in the *DSM-5-TR* (Norrholm et al., 2021; Pai et al., 2017). See Kilpatrick et al. (2013) for a discussion of the implications of this change.

Although the evaluator must always adhere to the current *DSM* criteria when making a diagnosis of medically related stress disorder, we suggest that the specifics of an adverse event be studied carefully in case a Criterion A trauma is actually present. For example, although COVID-19–related experiences often do not meet current criteria for a trauma designation, they would do so if the patient experienced "extreme anxiety/panic and fear of death during severe respiratory distress" (Norrholm et al., 2021, p. 1). Notably, even in cases in which a medical stressor does not rise to the level of a *DSM-5-TR* trauma, it can still underlie a variety of other disorders, including adjustment disorder, brief psychotic disorder with marked stressors, unspecified trauma- and stressor-related disorder, and some forms of depressive disorder.

Pregnancy and Infant Loss
Miscarriage occurs in up to 20% of all pregnancies (Blohm et al., 2008; Jeve & Davies, 2014), and stillbirth is estimated to occur in 1 of every 175 births in the United States (Gregory et al., 2023), with higher rates among racial and ethnic marginalized groups. Pregnancy and infant losses are widely experienced as traumatic, often resulting in sustained anxiety, grief, depression, posttraumatic stress, suicidality, or substance abuse (Farren et al., 2016; Weng et al., 2018). Effects are also found among partners of those who have miscarried (Due et al., 2017). Some people affected by pregnancy loss appear to recover within a year or two, whereas others may suffer for considerably longer (Janssen et al., 1997), especially those dealing with chronic infertility or previous miscarriages and stillbirths (Blackmore et al., 2011).

COVID-19
A dramatic example of medical trauma is the COVID-19 pandemic, which has resulted in widespread loss of life and a variety of serious and lasting health and mental health problems worldwide. In most cases, having severe COVID-19–related symptoms or being hospitalized for the disease would be insufficient to meet *DSM-5-TR* Criterion A for ASD or PTSD, even though the effects of COVID-19 infection often include symptoms consistent with posttraumatic stress (e.g., Bridgland et al., 2021).

Emergency Worker Trauma

First responders and other emergency personnel often encounter death, grotesque injury, and extreme victim distress. As a result, those who work with acutely traumatized people can become traumatized themselves. In fact, the *DSM-5-TR* trauma criteria refer to the experience of "repeated or extreme exposure to aversive details of the traumatic event(s)" (American Psychiatric Association, 2022, p. 301). Among those known to be at risk for such work-related traumas are firefighters, rescue workers, paramedics and other emergency medical personnel, emergency mental health workers, and law enforcement personnel (e.g., W. Berger et al., 2012; LaFauci Schutt & Marotta, 2011). Of late, extreme emotional distress has been documented in health care workers who were faced with unavoidable rationing and triage decisions during the COVID-19 pandemic (American Psychiatric Association, 2020).

Social Maltreatment

A strong case can be made that experiences of institutionalized maltreatment and oppression—such as racism, sexism, or discrimination against those identifying as LGBTQ+—constitute a major source of trauma for many in society (e.g., Allwood et al., 2022; Briere et al., 2025; Mooney, 2017). Social maltreatment can lead to acute distress, trigger painful memories of previous social maltreatment, exacerbate the effects of other traumas, and accumulate to produce lasting posttraumatic symptoms and responses (Briere et al., 2024; Nadal & Mendoza, 2014; Robinson & Rubin, 2016).

Microaggressions and Macroaggressions

Microaggressions, defined as "comment(s) or action(s) that subtly and often unconsciously or unintentionally express a prejudiced attitude toward a member of a marginalized group (such as a racial minority)" (Merriam-Webster, n.d.), can be acutely distressing and, as they accumulate, can lead to a range of negative psychological outcomes (Lui & Quezada, 2019; Sue et al., 2007). Macroaggressions, including hate crimes and related threats, stalking, bullying, and violence at the hands of authorities, are also obvious risk factors for psychological distress and disorder (Barnes & Ephross, 1994; Briere & Runtz, 2024).

Historical Trauma

Historical trauma can be defined as collective maltreatment by a dominant culture of a specific group of people that extends over generations. Examples of historical trauma in the United States include the enslavement of Black people for more than 250 years (DeGruy, 2017; Hannah-Jones, 2021); massacres, forced relocation, and near physical and cultural genocide of Native

Americans (Brave Heart & DeBruyn, 1998; Hartmann et al., 2019); and the widespread internment and maltreatment of people of Asian descent during and after World War II (Brockell, 2021; Nagata et al., 2019). Such adversities can have broad and ongoing social and cultural effects that are carried over the generations and tend to continue into the present in the form of systemic discrimination and social maltreatment.

Gender and Historical Trauma

Although those who identify as women and girls have often not been described as survivors of historical trauma, there is a centuries-long history of gender-based discrimination and victimization. Women and girls report higher rates of depression, anxiety, suicide attempts, PTSD, and eating disorders than men and boys (American Psychiatric Association, 2017; Briere & Scott, 2007; World Health Organization, 2000), which have been linked to their experience of more frequent sexual and domestic trauma throughout the lifespan, gender-based discrimination, restrictions on education and career advancement, and adverse gender socialization (e.g., Haahr-Pedersen et al., 2020; Rees et al., 2011; Silove et al., 2017; Vigod & Rochon, 2020).

Other Potentially Traumatic Adversities

Along with explicit experiences of maltreatment or victimization, there are adverse events or contexts that can be traumatizing by virtue of their inherent toxicity or because they increase the risk of victimization. These include the following:

- exposure to homelessness (Bassuk et al., 2001),
- extended poverty (Klest, 2012),
- living in communities characterized by violence and social marginalization (Fowler et al., 2009), and
- extended incarceration (Liem & Kunst, 2013).

Although they are generally not considered *DSM-5-TR*–level traumas, these adversities are associated with a range of negative outcomes, including posttraumatic stress (Ford et al., 2015, Chapter 11).

STRESSOR AND RESPONSE CHARACTERISTICS

Psychological outcomes following trauma exposure vary according to aspects of both the stressor itself and the response to that stressor, both within the individual and in the external environment. Both aspects of the stressor and the types of responses to stressors are discussed next.

Aspects of the Stressor

A number of stressor characteristics appear to affect posttraumatic outcome. Together, these characteristics are thought to reflect a general construct sometimes referred to as *stressor magnitude* or *stressor intensity*.

Variables that appear to increase stressor magnitude, and thus the likelihood or severity of PTSD or related outcomes, include the following:

- intentional acts of violence (as opposed to noninterpersonal events; e.g., Briere & Elliott, 2000);
- presence of life threat (e.g., DiGrande et al., 2011);
- physical injury (e.g., Foy et al., 1987);
- extreme or frequent combat exposure during war (e.g., Adams et al., 2016);
- witnessing death (e.g., C. J. Phillips et al., 2010), especially when grotesque in nature (e.g., R. S. Epstein et al., 1998);
- loss of a friend or loved one (e.g., Green et al., 1990);
- unpredictability and uncontrollability (e.g., Carlson & Dalenberg, 2000);
- sexual (as opposed to nonsexual) victimization (e.g., Kang et al., 2005); and
- traumas of longer duration, greater frequency, or greater complexity (Briere, Agee, et al., 2016; Courtois, 2004).

Although in many cases there appears to be a linear relationship between the extent or severity of the stressors and the subsequent posttraumatic response, this association is not especially large in magnitude and applies more to group data than to specific individuals. For example, it is not uncommon to encounter two people who experienced the same stressor (e.g., an earthquake or fire) who differ significantly in terms of their posttraumatic response. One individual may develop ASD, followed by PTSD, whereas another may experience few short-term or long-term effects. In addition, two stressors may appear objectively equivalent (e.g., two assaults of seemingly equal severity) yet have remarkably different effects on those involved.

Peritraumatic Responses

Emotional distress and dissociation—at the time of a trauma or immediately afterward—can affect an individual's internal experience and processing of the event. As a result, different types of peritraumatic responses can be associated with different posttraumatic outcomes.

Peritraumatic Distress

The trauma survivor's emotional response at the time of the potential stressor was given substantial credence by the *DSM-IV*, to the point that the negative event was not deemed a trauma if there was no report of concurrent horror, fear, or helplessness (Criterion A2). Although the *DSM-5-TR* PTSD criteria no longer include Criterion A2, there is little doubt that posttraumatic stress is more likely (and perhaps more intense) when the individual experiences one or more of these emotions peritraumatically (e.g., Brewin et al., 2000; Vance et al., 2018). Other negative emotional responses, such as anger, shame, and guilt, are also likely to increase the risk of posttraumatic reactions (e.g., Andrews et al., 2000; Bub & Lommen, 2017).

These findings imply that those who interpret a traumatic experience more negatively are at greater risk for posttraumatic difficulties, partially because of cognitive predispositions (e.g., the tendency to view life events as outside of one's control, or to perceive challenges as threats), partially as a function of preexisting stress intolerance, and partially because of the specific nature of the trauma (i.e., stressors vary according to the extent that they would motivate negative appraisal in most people). One individual may respond to an event with horror or helplessness because the event itself is horrific and overwhelming, whereas another might respond in a similar manner to a much lower magnitude stressor because of negative cognitive schema arising, for example, from previous child abuse experiences. To compound the complexity of subjective response, such attributions are almost always reported after the traumatic event and its effects have occurred (March, 1993). As a result, phenomena that occur after the event, such as the level of perceived support from others, subsequent negative or positive events, the effects of posttraumatic symptomatology, financial or interpersonal influences, or the results of professional intervention, are also important.

Peritraumatic Dissociation
Some research suggests that peritraumatic dissociative reactions (e.g., depersonalization or derealization around the time of the trauma) predict more extreme psychological outcomes, especially a greater likelihood of PTSD (e.g., Lensvelt-Mulders et al., 2008; Shalev et al., 1996). Such responses may interfere with the encoding and immediate processing of traumatic memories, thereby increasing the risk of more severe posttraumatic outcomes (e.g., Koopman et al., 1995). Although the correlation between peritraumatic dissociation and subsequent PTSD is substantial in some studies (Ozer et al., 2003), other researchers have failed to replicate this relationship (e.g., G. N. Marshall & Schell, 2002; Mellman et al., 2001) or report that the peritraumatic dissociation–PTSD connection disappears once other variables are taken into account (e.g., Holeva & Tarrier, 2001). In one study (Briere, Scott, et al., 2005), a measure of persistent and ongoing dissociation following a specific traumatic event was considerably more powerful in the prediction

of PTSD than was another scale measuring peritraumatic dissociative symptoms. In fact, peritraumatic dissociation ceased to be predictive of PTSD once sustained posttraumatic dissociation was taken into account through multiple regression analysis. These data suggest that whether one dissociates during a traumatic event may be less of a risk factor for PTSD than whether dissociation associated with the event (perhaps regardless of when it began) persists into the long term.

SOCIAL RESPONSE, SUPPORT, AND RESOURCES

As is especially reported in the interpersonal violence literature, posttraumatic states may vary in intensity as a function of the level of acceptance and support offered by others following the stressor. However, social response to the victim is not independent of trauma characteristics, victim variables, or environmental effects. Some traumatic events appear to be more socially acceptable than others. For example, a victim of a hurricane or earthquake may be seen as more innocent and worthy of compassion than a rape victim or someone targeted because of their sexual orientation. In addition, certain trauma survivors are more likely to receive prejudicial treatment than others, especially those living in poverty, members of racial and ethnic minority groups, those who identify as LGBTQ+, undocumented immigrants, women, people who have been trafficked or exploited (or both) by the sex industry, and those without housing (Bassuk et al., 2001; De Zulueta, 1998; Farley, 2004a; L. A. Goodman et al., 1991; Loo et al., 2001; West, 2002). This correlation between certain traumas, victims, and social variables may produce additional stigmatization and, as a result, reports of shame, guilt, or self-hatred (e.g., Hardesty & Greif, 1994; Herek et al., 1999).

Holding social prejudice constant, however, it appears that posttrauma support by family members, friends, helping professionals, and others can moderate the intensity of posttraumatic stress (Wang et al., 2021). Such support includes accepting (versus rejecting) responses after the trauma disclosure, nurturance from loved ones, an absence of stigmatization or blame by others, and availability of helpers and agencies after a traumatic experience. Importantly, Hobfoll (1988) noted that traumatic events not only produce stress, but they may also precipitate *loss spirals*, wherein the victim becomes more dependent on (and consuming of) social resources, eventually resulting in depletion of these resources, leading to additional stressors, greater vulnerability, and more stress responses. When the stressor affects an entire community (e.g., during a disaster), it may reduce social and physical resources at the same time that it traumatizes individuals, thereby producing more severe reactions (Norris & Thompson, 1995). When the stressor is more confined to the individual level (e.g., a rape or miscarriage), initial social support may decrease as the victim fails to recover in a time span expected by the social milieu, leading to victim perceptions of abandonment and rejection and, ultimately, potentially more severe stress responses.

CONCLUSION

The notion of what constitutes a traumatic event is less straightforward than might be envisioned. The initial intent of the *DSM-III* (American Psychiatric Association, 1980) was to define stressor characteristics, relatively independent of the victim, that were of sufficient intensity to produce a posttraumatic response in almost anyone. However, recent research suggests that the extent to which an event is traumatic is governed by the interaction between trauma magnitude and a range of victim variables that serve as relative risk factors for the development of posttraumatic stress. This interaction is further moderated by concurrent and postevent variables such as peritraumatic responses, level of social support and resources, cultural beliefs and expectations, and postevent attributions regarding the stressor.

It is clear that the interactionist view of traumatic events has lent greater precision to a clinical understanding of posttraumatic states. Among other things, this perspective increases the likelihood that the clinician will consider the stressor, the person, and their social network when evaluating the etiology of posttraumatic states. As has been found in other areas of mental health, the interactionist model suggests that posttraumatic stress rarely exists in a vacuum, and that the individual's responses to upsetting events must be considered within the context of their environment, resources, and life history.

On the other hand, the growing awareness of predisposing and moderating victim variables in PTSD response should not be used to discount the inherently traumatic nature of many events. Regardless of moderating victim and environmental phenomena, some events are intrinsically traumatic—acts of tremendous intrusion that negatively affect almost all of those who experience them. If these stressors are only considered traumatic when they produce a formal *DSM-5-TR* diagnosis of PTSD, there is a danger that the pain and lasting distress of many trauma survivors (e.g., those whose symptoms do not fit precisely into existing PTSD criteria) will be discounted. In contrast, the broader view of posttraumatic disturbance offered in the following chapters takes into account various types of disturbance, including subthreshold posttraumatic stress, ASD, complex PTSD, dissociation, and interpersonal sequelae, and thus implicates a wider range of potentially traumatic events.

2 TRAUMA-RELATED SYMPTOMS AND DISORDERS

There are a variety of posttraumatic outcomes, many of which are listed as disorders in the *Diagnostic and Statistical Manual of Mental Disorders, Fifth Edition, Text Revision* (*DSM-5-TR*; American Psychiatric Association, 2022). It should be reiterated, however, that not all trauma-related difficulties fit into specific diagnostic categories, in part because of the complex relationship between specific traumatic events and those individual and social variables outlined in the previous chapter. Trauma-related outcomes defy easy categorization. As a result, it is not always easy to define the clinical significance of a given person's posttraumatic disturbance based only on whether it meets the diagnostic criteria for a specific *DSM-5-TR* trauma-related disorder. This chapter describes two general types of trauma-related responses: those relatively specific to trauma exposure and those often (but not inevitably) associated with trauma.

TRAUMA- AND STRESS-SPECIFIC RESPONSES

The index diagnoses for extreme traumatization are often considered to be posttraumatic stress disorder (PTSD) or acute stress disorder (ASD), each of which is categorized as a trauma- and stressor-related disorder in the *DSM-5-TR*.

https://doi.org/10.1037/0000452-002
Psychological Assessment of Adult Posttraumatic States: *Phenomenology, Diagnosis, and Measurement, Third Edition*, by E. M. Eadie and J. Briere

This categorization of PTSD and ASD is a notable change from their designations as anxiety disorders in the fourth edition of the *DSM* (*DSM-IV*; American Psychiatric Association, 1994). Although these responses represent only a subset of the symptoms that can arise from trauma, they are quite prevalent among the trauma exposed. These diagnoses are discussed next.

Posttraumatic Stress Disorder

PTSD has been available as a diagnosis since the third edition of the *DSM* (*DSM-III*; American Psychiatric Association, 1980), although some version of its essential premise existed in the original *DSM* (*DSM-I*; gross stress reaction; American Psychiatric Association, 1952) and, to a considerably lesser extent, in the second edition (*DSM-II*; adjustment reaction of adult life; American Psychiatric Association, 1968). As *DSM* editions have evolved, both the definition of what it takes to produce PTSD (Chapter 1, this volume) and the symptoms associated with PTSD have changed as well. These developments have not been without controversy, however, and future *DSM* editions will no doubt further alter Criterion A and the symptoms thought to constitute PTSD.

Criterion A Revisited: Choice of Stressor in Measures of Posttraumatic Stress Disorder and Acute Stress Disorder

As will be described in Chapters 5 and 7, most trauma-relevant assessments can be divided into (a) those that require the respondent to report posttraumatic responses to a specific event (e.g., the Clinician-Administered PTSD Scale for *DSM-5* [CAPS-5]; F. W. Weathers, Blake, et al., 2013) and (b) those that make no reference to trauma exposure but instead investigate the frequency or severity of symptoms often associated with trauma (e.g., the Trauma Symptom Inventory–2 [TSI-2]; Briere, 2011). Although both approaches have benefits and drawbacks, neither actually parallels the *DSM-5-TR* option to link multiple different traumatic events to multiple different posttraumatic symptoms. In the latter instance, it is likely that the respondent will call upon recollections of multiple traumas and outcomes and, in this way, perhaps come closer to approximating the *DSM-5-TR* multiple trauma option. On the other hand, by not requiring any trauma specification, such tests may evaluate client responses to events that fall outside the purview of Criterion A—for example, major losses or relational breaches. As noted throughout this book, such non–Criterion A adversities are clearly worthy of assessment; however, they are not *DSM-5-TR* traumatic events, and any given diagnosis of PTSD (or ASD, as described in this chapter) generated by such a measure thus may be misleading.

The other common option, having the client pick a specific "index" trauma and then report all symptoms that explicitly arose from it, does ensure that a Criterion A event is being considered and thus that the prerequisite for a PTSD diagnosis has been met. However, this approach limits the respondent to symptoms arising from a single traumatic event even though the *DSM-5-TR* allows for a given instance of PTSD or ASD to arise from more than a single trauma. Furthermore, the lived reality of trauma for many people is that of multiple adverse events associated with a range of psychological symptoms and problems.

One possible solution to this conundrum is for the examiner to ask the client to rate their symptomatology separately for any number of specific traumas. For example, the CAPS *DSM-IV* interview (Blake et al., 1995) asked respondents to endorse up to three Criterion A events and to rate symptoms separately for each of these traumas. This approach can significantly extend the administration time of the diagnostic interview, however, and may still miss the effects of additional traumas (e.g., traumas 4 or 5 in a client with complex trauma exposure). Perhaps as a result, the CAPS-5 requires identification of a single index trauma, or multiple, closely related incidents, to serve as the basis of symptom inquiry (F. W. Weathers et al., 2018).

Symptomatology

As presented in Table 2.1, the symptoms of PTSD consist of four clusters:

- reexperiencing of the traumatic event,
- avoidance of trauma-relevant stimuli,
- numbing and negative cognitions and mood, and
- hyperarousal and hyperreactivity.

Reexperiencing involves flashbacks and intrusive thoughts or memories (or both) of the trauma, as well as distress and physiologic reactivity upon exposure to stimuli reminiscent of the event. *Avoidance* symptoms may be cognitive (e.g., avoiding upsetting thoughts, feelings, or memories) or behavioral (e.g., avoiding activities, people, places, or conversations that might trigger memories of the stressor). *Numbing* and *negative cognitions and mood* include diminished interest, detachment, and amnesia, as well as persistent negative beliefs and emotional states. The fourth PTSD symptom cluster, *hyperarousal and hyperreactivity*, often presents as jitteriness (jumpiness), irritability, sleep disturbance, self- or other-endangering behavior, angry outbursts, or attention or concentration difficulties.

As might be expected from the frequency of North Americans' exposure to traumatic events (Chapter 1, this volume), the lifetime prevalence of PTSD

TABLE 2.1. *DSM-5-TR* **Diagnostic Criteria for Posttraumatic Stress Disorder in Individuals Older Than 6 Years**

A. Exposure to actual or threatened death, serious injury, or sexual violence in one (or more) of the following ways:

  1. Directly experiencing the traumatic event(s).

  2. Witnessing, in person, the event(s) as it occurred to others.

  3. Learning that the traumatic event(s) occurred to a close family member or close friend. In cases of actual or threatened death of a family member or friend, the event(s) must have been violent or accidental.

  4. Experiencing repeated or extreme exposure to aversive details of the traumatic event(s) (e.g., first responders collecting human remains; police officers repeatedly exposed to details of child abuse).

  Note: Criterion A4 does not apply to exposure through electronic media, television, movies, or pictures, unless this exposure is work related.

B. Presence of one (or more) of the following intrusion symptoms associated with the traumatic event(s), beginning after the traumatic event(s) occurred:

  1. Recurrent, involuntary, and intrusive distressing memories of the traumatic event(s). **Note:** In children older than 6 years, repetitive play may occur in which themes or aspects of the traumatic event(s) are expressed.

  2. Recurrent distressing dreams in which the content and/or affect of the dream are related to the traumatic event(s). **Note:** In children, there may be frightening dreams without recognizable content.

  3. Dissociative reactions (e.g., flashbacks) in which the individual feels or acts as if the traumatic event(s) were recurring. (Such reactions may occur on a continuum, with the most extreme expression being a complete loss of awareness of present surroundings.)

  Note: In children, trauma-specific reenactment may occur in play.

  4. Intense or prolonged psychological distress at exposure to internal or external cues that symbolize or resemble an aspect of the traumatic event(s).

  5. Marked physiological reactions to internal or external cues that symbolize or resemble an aspect of the traumatic event(s).

C. Persistent avoidance of stimuli associated with the traumatic event(s), beginning after the traumatic event(s) occurred, as evidenced by one or both of the following:

  1. Avoidance of or efforts to avoid distressing memories, thoughts, or feelings about or closely associated with the traumatic event(s).

  2. Avoidance of or efforts to avoid external reminders (people, places, conversations, activities, objects, situations) that arouse distressing memories, thoughts, or feelings about or closely associated with the traumatic event(s).

D. Negative alterations in cognitions and mood associated with the traumatic event(s), beginning or worsening after the traumatic event(s) occurred, as evidenced by two (or more) of the following:

  1. Inability to remember an important aspect of the traumatic event(s) (typically due to dissociative amnesia and not to other factors such as head injury, alcohol, or drugs).

  2. Persistent and exaggerated negative beliefs or expectations about oneself, others, or the world (e.g., "I am bad," "No one can be trusted," "The world is completely dangerous," "My whole nervous system is permanently ruined").

TABLE 2.1. *DSM-5-TR* Diagnostic Criteria for Posttraumatic Stress Disorder in Individuals Older Than 6 Years (*Continued*)

   3. Persistent, distorted cognitions about the cause or consequences of the traumatic event(s) that lead the individual to blame himself/herself or others.

   4. Persistent negative emotional state (e.g., fear, horror, anger, guilt, or shame).

   5. Markedly diminished interest or participation in significant activities.

   6. Feelings of detachment or estrangement from others.

   7. Persistent inability to experience positive emotions (e.g., inability to experience happiness, satisfaction, or loving feelings).

E. Marked alterations in arousal and reactivity associated with the traumatic event(s), beginning or worsening after the traumatic event(s) occurred, as evidenced by two (or more) of the following:

   1. Irritable behavior and angry outbursts (with little or no provocation) typically expressed as verbal or physical aggression toward people or objects.

   2. Reckless or self-destructive behavior.

   3. Hypervigilance.

   4. Exaggerated startle response.

   5. Problems with concentration.

   6. Sleep disturbance (e.g., difficulty falling or staying asleep or restless sleep).

F. Duration of the disturbance (Criteria B, C, D, and E) is more than 1 month.

G. The disturbance causes clinically significant distress or impairment in social, occupational, or other important areas of functioning.

H. The disturbance is not attributable to the physiological effects of a substance (e.g., medication, alcohol) or another medical condition.

Specify whether:

   With dissociative symptoms: The individual's symptoms meet the criteria for posttraumatic stress disorder, and in addition, in response to the stressor, the individual experiences persistent or recurrent symptoms of either of the following:

   1. **Depersonalization:** Persistent or recurrent experiences of feeling detached from, and as if one were an outside observer of, one's mental processes or body (e.g., feeling as though one were in a dream; feeling a sense of unreality of self or body or of time moving slowly).

   2. **Derealization:** Persistent or recurrent experiences of unreality of surroundings (e.g., the world around the individual is experienced as unreal, dreamlike, distant, or distorted).

   Note: To use this subtype, the dissociative symptoms must not be attributable to the physiological effects of a substance (e.g., blackouts, behavior during alcohol intoxication) or another medical condition (e.g., complex partial seizures).

Specify if:

   With delayed expression: If the full diagnostic criteria are not met until at least 6 months after the event (although the onset and expression of some symptoms may be immediate).

Note. From *Diagnostic and Statistical Manual of Mental Disorders, Fifth Edition, Text Revision* (pp. 301–303), by the American Psychiatric Association, 2022. Copyright 2022 by the American Psychiatric Association. Reprinted with permission.

in the general population is significant. Several studies indicate that approximately 30% of individuals exposed to one or more Criterion A traumas will go on to experience PTSD (Santiago et al., 2013), and approximately 6% to 9% of North Americans will have experienced PTSD at some point in their lifetime (Goldstein et al., 2016; Kilpatrick et al., 2013). Most research suggests that women are approximately twice as likely as men to have PTSD at some point in their lifetime and, in the United States, African American individuals have higher rates than other racial groups (e.g., Kilpatrick et al., 2013; Roberts et al., 2011). Not surprisingly, individuals from countries that have undergone especially high levels of internal strife, violence, and war appear to have elevated rates of PTSD. For example, one major study reported estimated prevalences of PTSD (*DSM-IV*) of 37% in Algeria, 28% in Cambodia, 16% in Ethiopia, and 18% in Gaza (de Jong et al. 2001).

Acute Stress Disorder

According to the *DSM-5-TR*, "the essential feature of acute stress disorder is the development of characteristic symptoms lasting from 3 days to 1 month following exposure to one or more traumatic events" (American Psychiatric Association, 2022, p. 315). The specific symptoms of ASD are presented in Table 2.2.

ASD is noteworthy for its similarity to PTSD, except that it is diagnosed more acutely and there is no requirement that any given symptom be present; it only requires that a total of 9 or more of 14 symptoms be present. Importantly, although the *DSM-IV* required at least some dissociative symptoms, the *DSM-5-TR* no longer does so.

ASD is often a precursor to PTSD, including in the *DSM-IV* and *DSM-5* (American Psychiatric Association, 2013). For example, although a previous study reported that the *DSM-5* diagnostic criteria for ASD identified more patients with ASD (14%) than did the *DSM-IV* criteria (8%; Bryant et al., 2015), roughly equivalent proportions of people who were diagnosed with ASD went on to develop PTSD, irrespective of whether the *DSM-IV* or *DSM-5* criteria were used.

Individuals who experience acute stress reactions such as those listed for ASD sometimes present with psychomotor agitation or retardation, although these symptoms are not included in the *DSM-5-TR* criteria for ASD. Transient psychotic symptoms also may be present in some instances, especially when the stressor is severe or the victim is especially psychologically vulnerable. These symptoms may include cognitive loosening, briefly overvalued ideas or delusions, and hallucinations with trauma-related content.

TABLE 2.2. *DSM-5-TR* **Diagnostic Criteria for Acute Stress Disorder**

A. Exposure to actual or threatened death, serious injury, or sexual violence in one (or more) of the following ways:

   1. Directly experiencing the traumatic event(s).

   2. Witnessing, in person, the event(s) as it occurred to others.

   3. Learning that the event(s) occurred to a close family member or close friend. **Note:** In cases of actual or threatened death of a family member or friend, the event(s) must have been violent or accidental.

   4. Experiencing repeated or extreme exposure to aversive details of the traumatic event(s) (e.g., first responders collecting human remains, police officers repeatedly exposed to details of child abuse).

   Note: This does not apply to exposure through electronic media, television, movies, or pictures, unless this exposure is work related.

B. Presence of nine (or more) of the following symptoms from any of the five categories of intrusion, negative mood, dissociation, avoidance, and arousal, beginning or worsening after the traumatic event(s) occurred:

Intrusion Symptoms

   1. Recurrent, involuntary, and intrusive distressing memories of the traumatic event(s). **Note:** In children, repetitive play may occur in which themes or aspects of the traumatic event(s) are expressed.

   2. Recurrent distressing dreams in which the content and/or affect of the dream are related to the event(s). **Note:** In children, there may be frightening dreams without recognizable content.

   3. Dissociative reactions (e.g., flashbacks) in which the individual feels or acts as if the traumatic event(s) were recurring. (Such reactions may occur on a continuum, with the most extreme expression being a complete loss of awareness of present surroundings.) **Note:** In children, trauma-specific reenactment may occur in play.

   4. Intense or prolonged psychological distress or marked physiological reactions in response to internal or external cues that symbolize or resemble an aspect of the traumatic event(s).

Negative Mood

   5. Persistent inability to experience positive emotions (e.g., inability to experience happiness, satisfaction, or loving feelings).

Dissociative Symptoms

   6. An altered sense of the reality of one's surroundings or oneself (e.g., seeing oneself from another's perspective, being in a daze, time slowing).

   7. Inability to remember an important aspect of the traumatic event(s) (typically due to dissociative amnesia and not to other factors such as head injury, alcohol, or drugs).

Avoidance Symptoms

   8. Efforts to avoid distressing memories, thoughts, or feelings about or closely associated with the traumatic event(s).

   9. Efforts to avoid external reminders (people, places, conversations, activities, objects, situations) that arouse distressing memories, thoughts, or feelings about or closely associated with the traumatic event(s).

(continues)

TABLE 2.2. *DSM-5-TR* **Diagnostic Criteria for Acute Stress Disorder (*Continued*)**

Arousal Symptoms

    10. Sleep disturbance (e.g., difficulty falling or staying asleep, restless sleep).

    11. Irritable behavior and angry outbursts (with little or no provocation), typically expressed as verbal or physical aggression toward people or objects.

    12. Hypervigilance.

    13. Problems with concentration.

    14. Exaggerated startle response.

C. Duration of the disturbance (symptoms in Criterion B) is 3 days to 1 month after trauma exposure.

    Note: Symptoms typically begin immediately after the trauma, but persistence for at least 3 days and up to a month is needed to meet disorder criteria.

D. The disturbance causes clinically significant distress or impairment in social, occupational, or other important areas of functioning.

E. The disturbance is not attributable to the physiological effects of a substance (e.g., medication or alcohol) or another medical condition (e.g., mild traumatic brain injury) and is not better explained by brief psychotic disorder.

Note. From *Diagnostic and Statistical Manual of Mental Disorders, Fifth Edition, Text Revision* (pp. 313–315), by the American Psychiatric Association, 2022. Copyright 2022 by the American Psychiatric Association. Reprinted with permission.

When psychotic features are prominent, however, the appropriate diagnosis is usually brief psychotic disorder with marked stressors or, in some cases, major depressive disorder with psychotic features.

The prevalence of ASD (*DSM-5*) in the general population is not yet known. The incidence of ASD (*DSM-IV*) among traumatized individuals varies widely by study and trauma type. For example, motor vehicle accident victims have an approximately 13% chance of developing ASD (*DSM-IV*; Harvey & Bryant, 1998, 1999), whereas the rate for victims of interpersonal traumas is about 19% (Brewin et al. 1999). The *DSM-5-TR* cited research suggesting that less than 20% of individuals exposed to noninterpersonal traumas go on to develop ASD, whereas as many as 50% of those who experienced interpersonal traumas (e.g., assault or rape) may have symptoms that meet ASD criteria.

Regardless of whether ASD is different than PTSD on any dimension other than time of onset, and whatever its specific ability to predict later PTSD, it is a useful diagnosis for those experiencing severe symptoms immediately after a major accident, disaster, mass trauma, or interpersonal victimization. However, the decision to merely specify a range of symptoms that are equally relevant to ASD and PTSD may reduce the validity of this diagnosis. Because ASD may represent an early form of PTSD (Elklit & Brink, 2004), it seems logical that future *DSM* editions might settle on a common structure and set of diagnostic criteria.

Complex Posttraumatic Stress Disorder

Complex posttraumatic stress, also known as *complex PTSD* (Courtois & Ford, 2009; J. L. Herman, 1992a), is a relatively new addition to the trauma literature. Although complex PTSD is not listed in the *DSM-5 or DSM-5-TR*, it appears in the 11th edition of the *International Statistical Classification of Diseases and Related Health Problems (ICD-11*; Karatzias et al., 2017; World Health Organization, 2022). Complex PTSD, by definition, arises from exposure to complex trauma (Chapter 1, this volume) typically involving severe, prolonged, and repeated traumas and adversities, almost always of an interpersonal nature, typically beginning early in life and extending into adulthood (Briere & Scott, 2015; Ford & Courtois, 2020). Reflecting its chronic and often developmental etiology (for discussion of developmental trauma, refer to Chapter 1, this volume; also see Ford, 2021 and van der Kolk, 2005), this presentation often includes the somatic and dissociative problems described next, as well as chronic problems in identity (including self-esteem), boundary awareness, interpersonal relatedness, emotional regulation, and avoidance-focused behavior (Bachem et al., 2021; Ford & Courtois, 2020).

The relational and identity difficulties subsumed under complex PTSD reflect what Bachem and colleagues (2021) and the *ICD-11* refer to as *disturbances in self-organization* (DSOs). DSOs include the oft-cited tendency to be involved in chaotic and frequently maladaptive relationships, difficulty negotiating interpersonal boundaries, and reduced awareness of one's entitlements and needs in the presence of compelling others (Briere & Runtz, 2002; Cloitre et al., 2014). As noted earlier, this set of problems is often associated with a history of inadequate or disrupted caregiver–child attachment related to early childhood abuse, neglect, or parental disattunement (e.g., Godbout, Daspe, et al., 2019; Karatzias et al., 2021).

With some exceptions (e.g., Resick et al., 2012), most researchers currently agree that complex PTSD is a valid and discrete disorder (e.g., see Ford & Courtois, 2021; see also Cyr et al., 2022), albeit one whose internal structure may vary significantly as a function of gender or biological sex, neurobiology, age of onset, type and duration of trauma, early attachment disruption, and sociocultural factors.

Dissociative Disorders

The *DSM-5-TR* defines *dissociation* as "a disruption of and/or discontinuity in the normal integration of consciousness, memory, identity, emotion, perception, body representation, motor control and behavior" (American Psychiatric Association, 2022, p. 329). Central to most definitions is the notion of a variation in normal consciousness that arises from reduced or altered access to one's thoughts, feelings, perceptions, and/or memories, often in response to a traumatic event, that is not attributable to an underlying medical disorder (American Psychiatric Association, 2022; Brand et al., 2018; Cardeña & Carlson, 2011).

Although the phenomenology and etiology of dissociative responses has yet to be fully resolved, most studies report that dissociation is related to trauma (see reviews by Brand et al., 2018; Dalenberg et al., 2012; Loewenstein, 2018). Among the stressors associated with dissociation are child abuse (e.g., Dalenberg & Palesh, 2004), combat (e.g., Özdemir et al., 2015), sexual and physical assaults (e.g., Lipschitz et al., 1996; Schalinski et al., 2011), and natural disasters (Koopman et al., 1996).

Although dissociation is correlated with trauma exposure, this relationship is not as large as might be expected. For example, van Ijzendoorn and Schuengel (1996) reported that, across 26 studies, the average variance in Dissociative Experience Scale (E. M. Bernstein & Putnam, 1986) scores accounted for by participants' sexual or physical abuse history was 6%. Briere, Weathers, and Runtz (2005) found that respondents' lifetime history of trauma exposure accounted for an average of 4% of the variance in Multiscale Dissociation Inventory (Briere, 2002) subscale scores.

Above and beyond their frequent connection to trauma, some dissociative symptoms are associated with childhood experiences of neglect, parental disattunement, or early insecure parent–child attachment. Especially relevant may be the individual's early disorganized attachment to caregivers, involving chaotic, shifting, and intrusive responses to grossly confusing, fear-inducing, or painful parental behaviors, which may persist into the long term (Brand et al., 2022; Briere, Runtz, et al., 2019; Bureau et al., 2010).

This link to attachment might be taken to suggest that some dissociative symptoms are not trauma related. However, insecure attachment itself is often a trauma syndrome, as evidenced by the inclusion of attachment disorders in the *DSM-5-TR* "Trauma- and Stressor-Related Disorders" section. Attachment disruption often arises from negative events occurring very early in the child's life, as well as from acts of omission such as neglect, loss, or disattunement of such severity that it was terror inducing and developmentally disruptive (Ensink et al., 2020; Godbout, Daspe, et al., 2019). From this perspective, insecure attachment can be a marker for early, unreportable abuse, loss, or severe neglect, rather than an independent etiology.

Because dissociation is a frequent response to extreme stress, the clinician should consider dissociative symptoms and disorders as well as posttraumatic ones when assessing or treating trauma survivors. The dissociative disorders are described briefly next.

Depersonalization/Derealization Disorder

The *DSM-5-TR* defines the central feature of *depersonalization/derealization disorder* (DDD) as "clinically significant persistent or recurrent depersonalization (i.e., experiences of unreality or detachment from one's mind, self, or body) or derealization (i.e., experiences of unreality or detachment from one's surroundings)" while maintaining adequate reality testing (American Psychiatric Association, 2022, p. 329). The individual with DDD may feel like an automaton or robot, as if they are living in a movie, or like an outside observer of their mental processes or their body. Various types of sensory anesthesia, lack of emotional response, and a sensation of lacking control of one's actions may also be present, along with déjà vu experiences and perceptual distortions wherein objects or body parts appear to change shape or size. Sensory anesthesia often presents as feeling "dead" or "wooden."

Depersonalization and derealization disorder often arise from traumatic or highly stressful experiences (e.g., American Psychiatric Association, 2022; Murphy, 2023), although other etiologies, including traumatic brain injury, epilepsy, drug-related reactions, migraines, or panic attacks, are also possible (e.g., Lambert et al., 2002; R. D. Marshall et al., 2000). Traumas reported to produce depersonalization symptoms, or DDD, often include childhood maltreatment (King et al., 2020), but also motor vehicle accidents, disasters, and other immediately life-threatening experiences (e.g., American Psychiatric Association, 2022; Bryant & Harvey, 1999; Canan & North, 2019).

Dissociative Amnesia

The *DSM-5-TR* refers to *dissociative amnesia* as "an inability to recall autobiographical information that is inconsistent with normal forgetting" (American Psychiatric Association, 2022, p. 329). In the *DSM-III* and *DSM-III-R* (American Psychiatric Association, 1980, 1987), this disorder was named "psychogenic amnesia."

A review of medical journals published around the time of World War II suggested that psychogenic amnesia (then considered a symptom of hysteria) was a broadly accepted concept among combat physicians and was frequently documented in reports of war effects (e.g., Henderson & Moore, 1944; Sargant & Slater, 1941). More recently, traumatic events such as child abuse, torture, internment in concentration camps, physical assaults, motor vehicle accidents, and rape have been linked to reduced memory access (Courtois, 1999; Elliott, 1997; Loewenstein, 2018).

A number of studies of clinical and nonclinical research participants have found that either (a) a substantial proportion of those who report childhood trauma experiences (especially sexual abuse) also describe periods of partial or complete amnesia for said traumas (e.g., Elliott & Briere, 1995; M. A. Epstein & Bottoms, 2002; G. S. Goodman et al., 2003) or (b) some people with independently established histories of childhood sexual abuse will, on follow-up as adults, fail to report any memory of these experiences (e.g., L. M. Williams, 1994). Although there are problems with each of these studies, including, in some cases, retrospective reporting, lack of independent confirmation of self-reported trauma history, and the potential confounding of amnesia with reluctance to disclose (Berliner & Briere, 1998; Mangiulli et al., 2021), it seems unlikely that all of them misidentify lack of trauma-related memories as amnesia. In support of the likelihood that at least some trauma memories are inaccessible to some survivors, functional magnetic resonance imaging research indicates specific neural systems associated with blocking unwanted memories from consciousness (Anderson et al., 2004), including reduced activity of the amygdala and increased activity of the prefrontal cortex among those with dissociative amnesia (for review, see Kendall, 2021).

Notably, the probable existence of trauma-specific amnesia does not rule out the possibility of confabulated ("false") memory (Lindsay & Briere, 1997). As the *DSM-5-TR* noted, "there is no test, battery of tests, or set of procedures that invariably distinguishes dissociative amnesia from feigned amnesia" (American Psychiatric Association, 2022, p. 342). As a result, the clinician must approach any given report of memory recovery (or any other uncorroborated historical statement) with care, neither ruling in nor ruling out such reports without due consideration of all relevant information.

Dissociative Identity Disorder

Probably the least common of the dissociative disorders is *dissociative identity disorder* (DID). The *DSM-5-TR* diagnostic criteria for DID refer to a "disruption of identity characterized by two or more distinct personality states" involving a "marked discontinuity in sense of self and sense of agency, accompanied by related alterations in affect, behavior, consciousness, memory, perception, cognition, and/or sensory-motor functioning" (American Psychiatric Association, 2022, p. 330).

Although the *DSM-5-TR* specifies "two or more distinct personality states" in the criteria for DID, it is not uncommon for individuals with a diagnosis of DID to report a greater number of discrete identities as well as less coherent personality fragments (International Society for the Study of Trauma and Dissociation, 2011; Putnam et al., 1986). Patients with DID often report an amnestic barrier between at least some identities, such that one personality state may have little or no knowledge of the existence of other personality states (Spiegel et al., 2011).

Of the various disorders, DID has been most frequently linked to extreme maltreatment during childhood, especially sexual or physical abuse (Loewenstein, 2018). Other childhood traumas implicated in DID include experiencing the death or loss of a significant other and witnessing the intentional killing of another or others (Kluft, 1993).

The diagnosis of DID is relatively controversial in mental health circles. Some question the validity of DID as a naturally occurring phenomenon, dispute the connection between DID and child abuse, or suggest that some cases are iatrogenically associated with suggestibility during treatment, fantasy proneness, or exposure to mass media coverage of the issue (see discussions by Brand et al., 2018; Loewenstein, 2018). Although this issue is unlikely to be resolved to all parties' satisfaction, research over the last several decades suggests that DID (a) can occur as a natural psychological phenomenon, albeit potentially a relatively rare one; (b) usually arises from extended and extreme childhood trauma; and (c) is sometimes misrepresented as present or absent in the context of poorly conducted psychological assessment or treatment (Dalenberg et al., 2020).

Brief Psychotic Disorder With Marked Stressors

Brief psychotic disorder with marked stressors (BPDMS) appeared in the *DSM-III-R* as "brief reactive psychosis" (American Psychiatric Association, 1987). In later *DSM* editions, the focus has been on the chronology of the disorder, not its etiology. As a result, the clinician can apply the brief psychotic disorder diagnosis when there is no stressor (i.e., brief psychotic disorder without marked stressors) or where stressors exist (i.e., BPDMS). There also is an option to diagnose brief psychotic disorder with postpartum onset. In the case of marked stressors, the precipitating event is generally equivalent to those included in Criterion A of ASD or PTSD, although the *DSM-5-TR*, stating that "psychotic symptoms occur in response to events that, singly or together, would be markedly stressful to almost anyone in similar circumstances in the individual's culture," is less specific here and more reminiscent of the *DSM-III* (American Psychiatric Association, 1980, p. 109). Traumas linked to BPDMS in the literature include severe accidents, major losses, assaults, and disasters (American Psychiatric Association, 2022). Notably, individuals with preexisting psychotic symptomatology are often at greater risk of subsequent interpersonal violence (de Vries et al., 2019), sometimes making it difficult to discriminate whether a given trauma is etiological or an epiphenomenon of vulnerability to maltreatment.

BPDMS is noteworthy for the fact that the psychotic episode often begins abruptly and may be quite florid in nature. The diagnosis requires at least one of four psychotic symptoms (delusions, hallucinations, disorganized speech, or grossly disorganized or catatonic behavior), although several are usually present simultaneously. Like other acute psychotic phenomena, BPDMS is sometimes accompanied by extreme agitation, emotional distress, and confusion. The *DSM-5-TR* lists suicide attempts as an associated feature, and it notes that those with this disorder may require close supervision. The duration of BPDMS ranges from 1 day to less than 1 month, with eventual return to premorbid functioning.

It is not always clear whether a psychotic episode that follows a traumatic stressor is, in fact, BPDMS. As noted in the *DSM-IV-TR*, in some cases the psychosis may appear to be trauma related but persist for several months or longer (American Psychiatric Association, 2000, pp. 330–331). Unfortunately, because such symptoms exceed the (somewhat arbitrary) 1-month limit, they cannot be diagnosed as BPDMS but instead must be diagnosed as some other (nonstressor-related) psychotic disorder. In other instances, psychotic responses to a marked stressor may represent the activation of a latent predisposition toward psychosis or the acute exacerbation of an already existing—but previously undetected—psychotic illness, such as schizophrenia, schizophreniform disorder, or a delusional disorder.

It also is not uncommon for a severe trauma to produce or trigger a psychotic depression, as noted later in this chapter—a diagnosis that takes precedence over BPDMS. Finally, as noted earlier, some instances of severe posttraumatic stress may include psychotic symptoms (e.g., paranoid ideation, looseness of thought, or hallucinations) in the context of a more prominent ASD or PTSD presentation (Compean & Hamner, 2019). For example, it has been estimated that 30% to 40% of treatment-seeking Vietnam War combat veterans with PTSD experience at least some hallucinations or delusions (David et al., 1999), and research on the more severe and complex effects of child abuse suggests that some psychotic symptoms can arise from early childhood trauma and maltreatment (Read et al., 2001).

SYMPTOMS AND DISORDERS OFTEN RELATED TO TRAUMA EXPOSURE OR ANOTHER MAJOR STRESSOR

Two additional diagnoses are relevant in the presence of exposure to a trauma or a major stressor: adjustment disorder (AD) and prolonged grief disorder (PGD). Although not all instances of these disorders arise from a *DSM-5-TR* trauma per se, they are not uncommon among individuals exposed to extreme adversity. As a result, AD and PGD are now included in the *DSM-5-TR* "Trauma- and Stressor-Related Disorders" section and in the *ICD-11* "Disorders Specifi- cally Associated with Stress" section.

Adjustment Disorder

The *DSM-5-TR* diagnosis of AD involves the development of clinically signifi- cant emotional or behavioral (but not normal bereavement) symptoms within 3 months of exposure to an identifiable stressor, as evidenced by either (a) marked distress that is greater than—or out of proportion to—what would be expected by exposure to the stressor or (b) significant impairment in social, occupational, or other important areas of functioning. The *DSM-5-TR* adds the proviso that cultural and contextual factors should be considered before stressor-related symptoms can be considered sufficiently out of proportion to warrant an AD diagnosis.

The *DSM-5-TR* notes that a diagnosis of AD cannot be made if symptoms meet the criteria for another *DSM* disorder or represent an exacerbation of a preexisting disorder. AD is specified as *acute* if the symptoms last less than 6 months or *chronic* if they last longer. The subtypes of AD are as follows:

- with anxiety,
- with depressed mood,
- with disturbance of conduct,
- with mixed anxiety and depressed mood,
- with mixed disturbance of emotions and conduct, and
- unspecified.

AD is relatively common among clinical samples, people who are unemployed, medical patients, and bereaved individuals (e.g., O'Donnell et al., 2019). In a study of more than 800 hospitalized patients with injury, 19% were diag- nosed with AD (*DSM-5*) at 3 months after trauma versus 16% at 12 months, and classical PTSD symptoms were common at both time intervals (O'Donnell et al., 2016). O'Donnell and colleagues (2016) noted that AD did not appear to be a stable disorder, as "two-thirds of those who had the disorder at 3 months no longer had the diagnosis at 12 months" (p. 1236).

Because of the range of adverse events potentially associated with AD, this diagnosis can be used when the stressor falls short of ASD/PTSD Criterion A (e.g., divorce, a serious [but not life-threatening] medical condition, financial difficulties, or being fired from one's job). In addition, the hallmark symptoms of AD typically are sustained dysphoria or maladaptive behavior, as opposed to the specific reliving, avoidant, and hyperarousal symptoms most characteristic of PTSD. It should be noted, however, that the diagnosis can be applied in cases in which there was a PTSD-level trauma and the symptoms arising from it do not meet criteria for any other, more specific disorder. When the differential diagnosis involves high-level (i.e., Criterion A) stressors, three questions should be asked, in the following order:

1. Are the symptoms best described as a classic stress disorder or another condition? If yes, consider *ASD, PTSD, BPDMS*, and so on.

2. If no to question 1, do the symptoms involve subthreshold posttraumatic stress? If yes, consider *other specified/or unspecified trauma- and stressor-related disorders*.

3. If no to question 2, have the symptoms been present within 6 months of the offset of the stressor, and do they appear to be something other than a normal grief reaction? If yes, consider *AD*.

Grief

Grief is a normal response to loss and often resolves naturally over time. When the loss involves a sudden, traumatic, or even violent death or disruption of an individual's life, however, this response may become more complicated and may be associated with lasting health and mental health problems and reduced response to treatment (N. M. Simon et al., 2020). For example, traumatic loss may be accompanied by clinical depression, posttraumatic stress, substance abuse, psychosis, or, in some cases, serious physical illness (Shear & Smith-Caroff, 2002; Van Ommeren et al., 2001). A "complicated" or "traumatic" grief disorder following traumatic loss was suggested in the late 1990s (Prigerson et al., 1999), a version of which was included as a condition for further study in the *DSM-5*. The suggested persistent complex bereavement disorder had a specifier, with traumatic bereavement, to be used when the symptoms of bereavement include "persistent distressing preoccupations regarding the traumatic nature of the death (often in response to loss reminders)" (American Psychiatric Association, 2013, p. 790).

Ultimately, the *DSM-5* committee decided not to include bereavement as a separate disorder, but rather eliminated the *DSM-IV* bereavement exclusion for major depressive disorder that had previously kept clinicians from diagnosing depression if it arose in response to grief. With the *DSM-5* criteria, individuals with grief-related depression that lasts for more than 2 weeks can be diagnosed with major depression.

Prolonged Grief Disorder

In light of research suggesting that extended grief responses differ in significant ways from general depression, the *DSM-5-TR* (American Psychiatric Association, 2022) introduced a new diagnosis, *prolonged grief disorder*, which discriminates extended grief from both depression and posttraumatic stress. Notably, the diagnosis of PGD can only be made after a year of symptoms and emphasizes extended and unresolved yearning for the deceased, loss of meaning, and identity disruption (Prigerson et al., 2021). Given the 1-year requirement and the fact that the diagnostic criteria are not focused on trauma per se, PGD is, unfortunately, less relevant to more acute grief responses, which are instead typically subsumed under the diagnosis of major depression.

GENERIC SYMPTOMS AND DISORDERS OFTEN RELATED TO TRAUMA EXPOSURE OR ANOTHER MAJOR STRESSOR

The disorders discussed next highlight the importance of assessing for trauma exposure when evaluating any anxiety, mood, psychotic, or other disorder. Although assessments of PTSD, ASD, and even AD require exposure to a qualifying trauma or stressor for the diagnosis to be made, many assessing clinicians do not sufficiently assess for trauma exposure as they evaluate the presence and extent of other disorders, despite the relevance to overall conceptualization and understanding of an individual.

Anxiety

Anxiety symptoms are a feature of traumatic stress disorders (e.g., hypervigilance, physiological reactions to trauma cues), and some anxiety disorders are triggered or exacerbated by exposure to a traumatic event. Prior to publication of the *DSM-5*, PTSD and ASD were, in fact, categorized in the "Anxiety Disorders" section before being moved to the new "Trauma- and Stressor-Related Disorders" section. This highlights the fear-based components of trauma reactions and the historical understanding of significant overlap between anxiety disorders and traumatic stress disorders.

Generalized Anxiety Disorder

Generalized anxiety disorder (GAD) is both a risk factor for developing posttraumatic stress in response to a trauma (Koenen et al., 2002) and a syndrome that may follow trauma exposure (Ayazi et al., 2014). In the *DSM-5-TR*, the symptoms of GAD involve the following:

- Excessive anxiety and worry (apprehensive expectation), occurring more days than not for at least 6 months, about a number of events or activities (such as work or school performance);

- Trouble controlling such worry; and

- At least three of six specific symptoms:

  −restlessness,

  −being easily fatigued,

  −concentration problems,

  −irritability,

  −muscle tension, or

  −sleep disturbance. (American Psychiatric Association, 2022, p. 250)

Because anxiety is probably a final common pathway for a variety of etiological factors, some of which are not trauma related, the presence of generalized anxiety in any given individual does not necessarily mean that they have a trauma history. In traumatized individuals, however, such nonspecific anxiety often reflects the impact of upsetting or threatening events in the past.

Panic Disorder

Although panic disorder is not traditionally considered trauma related, the *DSM-5-TR* notes that panic attacks can arise from loss or disruption of important interpersonal relationships and suggests a possible link between panic disorder and posttraumatic stress (American Psychiatric Association, 2022, pp. 238–239). In fact, the *DSM-5-TR* states that between 10% and 60% of individuals with panic disorder report a history of trauma (p. 239). In a direct investigation of panic and trauma exposure, Falsetti and Resnick (1997) found that 69% of clients seeking treatment for trauma-related symptomatology reported trauma-specific panic attacks. In addition, various investigators (e.g., Kellner & Yehuda, 1999; Southwick et al., 1997) suggested that panic disorder and PTSD may involve hyperactivation of similar neurobiological (e.g., noradrenergic or serotonergic) circuits in the brain.

These data suggest that panic can be a posttraumatic stress response, although not all panic attacks arise from traumatic events. When panic is trauma related, several etiologic pathways are possible. First, panic attacks may arise from the inescapable fear associated with some traumas, and thus may represent a classically conditioned response that can be activated by stimuli reminiscent of the original traumatic event. Second, panic episodes may arise from the experience of PTSD, wherein repeated flashbacks, along with autonomic hyperarousal, activate anticipatory fear responses. Finally, traumatic exposure likely enhances or kindles reactivity of the sympathetic nervous system (e.g., Lissek & van Meurs, 2015), making panic symptoms (and panic disorder) more likely.

Despite the link between panic and PTSD, the *DSM-5-TR* notes that panic attacks cannot be considered evidence of panic disorder if they are specifically triggered by recollections or reminders of a traumatic event. Thus, for example, a rape survivor's panic attack on seeing someone similar to their assailant might be considered an associated feature of PTSD if they had that disorder, but it would not be categorized as a symptom of panic disorder. If, however, after the rape, the survivor began having unexpected panic attacks in a situation that did not trigger rape memories, panic disorder might be a relevant diagnosis.

Phobic Anxiety

Most perspectives on the etiology of irrational fears (i.e., phobias) stress conditioned fear responses to stimuli associated with prior upsetting events, although some also note genetic aspects of phobia development (e.g., Kendler et al., 2002). In line with conditioning theory, many of the avoidant symptoms of PTSD and ASD are implicitly phobic, involving efforts to avoid people, places, and situations that are reminiscent of a given trauma. Phobias have been found to be more prevalent among individuals exposed to trauma and are sometimes comorbid with posttraumatic stress (Carleton et al., 2011; Cougle et al., 2010).

Depression

When posttraumatic and depressive symptoms arise from the same or related traumas, survivors often report grief and loss, abandonment, and isolation. The overlap between posttraumatic stress, grief, and depression described earlier, as well as the connection between depression and heightened suicide potential in trauma survivors (e.g., Briere, Kwon, et al., 2019; Briere, Madni, & Godbout, 2016; Ogata et al., 2011), suggests that depression should always be considered when assessing those who have been traumatized.

Major Depression

Various studies report that those who have been exposed to a major trauma are at risk of developing major depressive disorder. In fact, depression is one of the most common comorbid disorders for PTSD (e.g., El Baba & Colucci,

2018; Kessler et al., 1995). Certain symptoms of depression (particularly insomnia, psychomotor agitation, loss of interest in formerly enjoyable events, and decreased ability to concentrate) overlap with symptoms of PTSD (Gros et al., 2010), which may complicate assessment. Additionally, some trauma survivors present with a chief complaint of depressed mood but do not initially report a trauma history. As a result, clinicians evaluating trauma survivors should be alert to depressive symptoms, including the following:

- extreme sadness related to irrevocable loss;
- hopelessness regarding the likelihood of future traumatic events;
- feelings of worthlessness, excessive guilt, or thoughts about having deserved a traumatic event;
- suicidality;
- loss of interest in formerly pleasurable activities;
- reduced ability to concentrate;
- psychomotor agitation or retardation;
- anorexia and/or weight gain or loss;
- fatigue and loss of energy; and
- sleep disturbance, either insomnia or hypersomnia.

A number of clinicians and researchers have noted a tendency for posttraumatic and depressive symptoms to arise from the same stressor (e.g., Pickens et al., 1995; Yehuda et al., 1994). In addition, studies indicate significant comorbidity between PTSD and depression (Armenta et al., 2019; Flory & Yehuda, 2015; O'Donnell et al., 2004). Although neither literature proves the existence of posttraumatic depression per se, both suggest that events severe enough to produce posttraumatic stress can also produce or exacerbate depressive symptoms. Posttraumatic depression does not appear as a specific diagnosis in the *DSM-5-TR*, however.

Major Depression With Psychotic Features
Given the relationship between PTSD and both depression and psychosis, it is not surprising that major depression with psychotic features also has been linked to posttraumatic stress. More unexpected is the fact that PTSD is more common among depressed individuals with psychotic symptoms than among depressed individuals without psychosis. For example, in a sample of 500 psychiatric outpatients, Zimmerman and Mattia (1999) found that those with psychotic depression were nearly four times more likely to have PTSD than those with nonpsychotic depression (58% vs. 16%). Such data align with findings that among those with PTSD, psychotic symptoms are often comorbid with major depression (e.g., R. S. Wilson et al., 2020).

The elevated risk of PTSD in individuals with psychotic depression may be explained in several ways. First, it may be that extreme trauma produces both psychosis and depression, such that some individuals present with both sets of symptoms simultaneously. Second, those with a predisposition to psychotic depression may be at risk for PTSD by virtue of decreased emotional regulation abilities or a tendency to become cognitively disorganized when stressed. Third, some of the psychotic symptoms experienced by PTSD sufferers with comorbid depression may reflect severe intrusive or dissociative symptomatology associated with posttraumatic stress. For example, hearing voices is not uncommon among individuals exposed to trauma (Shinn et al., 2019). Regardless of the reasons for the associations among posttraumatic stress, depression, and psychosis, the assessing clinician (a) should be alert to the possibility of significant trauma exposure in those who complain both of psychotic and depressive symptoms and (b) should be prepared to discriminate between these conditions when they overlap or mimic each other.

Substance Use

Problematic substance use is common among individuals exposed to trauma, especially those who have experienced interpersonal violence (Ford & Hawke, 2015; Hedtke et al., 2008), and those with substance use problems are more likely than those in many other groups to report symptoms of PTSD (e.g., Ullman et al., 2013). Chilcoat and Breslau (1998) found that individuals with PTSD were four times more likely to excessively use alcohol or drugs than those without PTSD, irrespective of trauma history, whereas substance use was not a predictor of subsequent trauma exposure or PTSD in that study. Nevertheless, some research suggests that major substance use increases the likelihood of interpersonal victimization (e.g., Logan et al., 2002) and exposure to automobile accidents (Ursano et al., 1999).

There are at least three major reasons why trauma, PTSD, and substance use might overlap (Briere, 2019; P. J. Brown & Wolfe, 1994):

- trauma survivors may seek out psychoactive substances to numb or distract from posttraumatic distress,

- those who heavily use substances are more easily victimized and are more likely to be involved in accidents, and

- major substance use can exacerbate or increase the risk of symptomatology (e.g., PTSD) in those exposed to trauma.

Distress Reduction Behaviors

Sometimes seen as symptoms of borderline personality disorder (BPD), impulse control disorder, or a behavioral addiction, there are a number of seemingly dysfunctional or self-defeating behaviors that are common among those with childhood histories of abuse, neglect, or insecure attachment. They include the following:

- deliberate, but nonsuicidal, self-injury (e.g., Briere & Eadie, 2016);
- triggered suicidal behavior (e.g., Pezawas et al., 2002);
- risky or compulsive sexual behavior (e.g., Vaillancourt-Morel et al., 2015);
- food bingeing and purging (e.g., Rosenbaum & White, 2013);
- compulsive gambling (American Psychiatric Association, 2013);
- compulsive shoplifting (American Psychiatric Association, 2013);
- reactive aggression (e.g., Fite et al., 2009);
- compulsive skin picking and hair pulling (e.g., Stein et al., 2010);
- fire setting (e.g., Blanco et al., 2010); and
- extensive preoccupation with Internet activities (e.g., Charlton & Danforth, 2007).

These symptoms are referred to as *distress reduction behaviors* (DRBs; Briere, 2019) because they appear to reflect attempts to distract, numb, block, counteract, or otherwise avoid distress associated with triggered abuse or attachment memories, generally in the context of reduced or unavailable emotional regulation capacities. DRBs, a form of behavioral avoidance, are thought to arise when painful childhood memories (including preverbal schema arising from early attachment breaches or insecurity) are triggered by current relational stimuli that, in the absence of sufficient emotional regulation skills, are overwhelming and motivate avoidance. In support of this perspective, each of the DRBs just listed has been associated with antecedent childhood abuse or neglect, attachment disturbance, or decreased emotional regulation capacities (Briere, 2019).

Research and clinical practice suggest that DRBs provide one or more of the following psychological functions:

- distraction from painful internal states,
- self-soothing,
- interruption of unwanted numbing or dissociation,
- distress-incompatible experiences,
- momentary interpersonal connection,
- self-punishment to reduce guilt or shame,
- communication of emotional distress in the face of social disconnection, and

- an increased sense of control (e.g., Briere & Eadie, 2016; Klonsky, 2007; Yates, 2004).

It is important to note that DRBs are associated with some instances of BPD (described next) but are not pathognomonic indicators of that disorder, with many DRB-involved clients not meeting criteria for BPD and not all BPD sufferers necessarily engaging in DRBs (Briere, 2019; Briere & Scott, 2015).

Borderline Personality Disorder

The *DSM-5-TR* describes BPD as a chronic disturbance in which there is "a pervasive pattern of instability of interpersonal relationships, self-image, and affects, and marked impulsivity, beginning by early adulthood and present in a variety of contexts" (American Psychiatric Association, 2022, p. 752). The symptoms of BPD include the following:

- "frantic" attempts to avoid perceived abandonment by others;
- unstable interpersonal relationships;
- identity disturbance;
- potentially self-endangering impulsivity;
- suicidality or self-injurious behavior;
- emotional instability;
- feelings of emptiness;
- inappropriate, intense anger; and
- episodes of stress-related paranoia or severe dissociation.

BPD, its presumed etiology, and its defining symptoms have gone through many iterations. Most modern perspectives link this disorder to severe childhood abuse, neglect, and disattunement and associated insecure attachment (e.g., Briere & Scott, 2015; Hailes et al., 2019; van Dijke et al., 2012). Also implicated are neurobiological irregularities frequently associated with trauma exposure, including in the hippocampus, frontal cortex, amygdala, and hypothalamic-pituitary-adrenal (HPA) axis (Driessen et al., 2000; N. Thomas et al., 2019).

In a structural equation model analysis of a large nonclinical sample, Godbout et al. (2019) found that childhood trauma and attachment predictors of BPD-related symptomatology may vary as a function of the gender of participants and of their abusive or neglectful parents. In women, child maltreatment by both mothers and fathers appeared to be directly associated with borderline symptoms; in men, only maltreatment by fathers was so related. The effects of attachment history on borderline symptoms varied according to gender, with women maltreated by fathers being indirectly associated with symptoms via insecure attachment; in men, maltreatment by mothers indirectly predicted symptoms of BPD via insecure attachment.

The construct validity of BPD is subject to considerable theoretical debate (e.g., Lewis & Grenyer, 2009; New et al., 2008), with some questioning whether it is a specific disorder. Some researchers and clinicians, for example, suggest that what is referred to as BPD is a heterogeneous collection of symptoms and problems that vary according to a wide range of factors and that overlap with several other disorders—including those related to trauma, emotional dysregulation, and attachment disturbance (Brand & Lanius, 2014; Briere & Scott, 2015; Kulkarni, 2017).

An active debate in the literature is whether what appears to be BPD is, in fact, complex PTSD as described earlier. However, multivariate analyses (e.g., see Cloitre et al., 2014; Cyr et al., 2022) suggest that BPD, complex PTSD, and PTSD are all related to trauma exposure but are likely different entities (see discussion by Ford & Courtois, 2021). These findings further suggest that BPD may represent a real phenomenon, albeit not the one that earlier clinicians presumed. BPD may best be seen as a multidimensional phenomenon that involves identity problems, emotional dysregulation, DRBs, and interpersonal dysfunction that has not been adequately characterized to date and is related to gender, type of child maltreatment, parental disattunement, insecure attachment, and altered neurobiology. Notably, this complex version should not be confused with historically defined BPD, which relies on outmoded etiological and phenomenological models and tends to be stigmatizing (Aviram et al., 2006).

Psychosis

Psychotic symptoms (hallucinations, delusions, tangential or loosened mental associations, and some instances of catatonic behavior) are not only present in schizophrenia and other psychotic disorders; as indicated previously, they may also follow exposure to overwhelmingly traumatic events (Hardy & Mueser, 2017). For example, a significant number of treatment-seeking Vietnam War combat veterans with PTSD experience at least some hallucinations or delusions (or both; e.g., David et al., 1999), and psychotic symptoms have been reported by assault survivors (Kilcommons et al., 2008) and those who were maltreated as children (Bebbington et al., 2011). Childhood trauma and abuse is often associated with more severe and varied psychotic symptoms and more disturbed behavior (Álvarez et al., 2011), and it may influence the content of psychotic delusions and hallucinations (Bentall et al., 2012).

Notably, some seemingly psychotic symptoms, such as catatonia or hallucinations, may actually reflect trauma-related dissociative symptomatology, potentially leading to instances when a dissociative disorder (perhaps especially DID) is misdiagnosed as a psychotic one (Brand, 2024; H. Hall, 2024). Furthermore, dissociation can be comorbid with, or an associated feature of, some psychotic presentations (Fung et al., 2024; Longden et al., 2020). As a result, it is important that the assessor evaluate the presence or absence of dissociative symptoms that may mimic or accompany psychosis (Brand, 2024; Longden et al., 2020).

Schizophrenia

It has been assumed that the most common psychotic disorder, schizophrenia, does not have a significant connection to trauma. Instead, schizophrenia is often viewed as arising from genetic factors, with elevated rates found among identical twins and siblings whose parents suffer from schizophrenia (for review, see Sullivan, 2005). Recent studies and analyses, however, implicate trauma, especially severe childhood abuse (for review, see Popovic et al., 2019). For example, a meta-analysis of 20 studies of the relationship between schizophrenia and childhood abuse (Morgan & Fisher, 2007) found that 50% of people with schizophrenia, across gender, had experienced sexual or physical abuse.

These studies do not mean that schizophrenia necessarily arises directly from childhood trauma exposure, however. Some hallucinations identified in trauma survivors may be posttraumatic flashbacks, some delusions may involve trauma-based cognitive distortions and hypervigilance, and some of the seemingly negative signs of schizophrenia may reflect numbing or posttraumatic dissociation. Nevertheless, given the neural diathesis-stress model of schizophrenia (Jones & Fernyhough, 2007), some individuals who ultimately manifest schizophrenic symptoms may do so because a genetic predisposition to schizophrenia is activated by the stressful effects of childhood trauma. It is also possible that a neurodevelopmental interaction between the biology of posttraumatic stress—for example, alterations in the HPA axis, prefrontal cortex, and amygdala—influences the development of at least some instances of schizophrenia (Popovic et al., 2019; Read et al., 2001).

PHYSICAL OR MEDICAL SYMPTOMS

Symptoms that present in the body are common in many psychological disorders (e.g., depression, generalized anxiety). When physical or medical symptoms are among the primary complaints, diagnoses under the new *DSM-5* category, "Somatic Symptom and Related Disorders," should be considered. Individuals with these concerns often first present to primary care practitioners rather than mental health professionals. Thus, it is especially important for history of trauma exposure and related posttraumatic states to also be investigated if a somatic presentation of psychological distress is suspected.

Somatic Symptom Disorder

Somatic symptom disorder (SSD) consists of a wide variety of symptoms, the only commonality of which seems to be their somatic focus and the fact that they either cannot be explained medically or that their intensity is beyond that expected from their medical etiology. This disorder is diagnosed when the individual "has a significant focus on physical symptoms, such as pain, weakness or shortness of breath, to a level that results in major distress and/or problems functioning. . . . The physical symptoms may or may not be associated with a diagnosed medical condition" (American Psychiatric Association, 2024, para. 1).

Per the *DSM*-5 and *DSM-5-TR*, the severity of SSD depends on whether there are a wide variety of physical symptoms (in the severe form) or just one or two (mild or moderate forms, respectively). SSD symptoms have been associated with child abuse and later trauma in several studies (e.g., Kealy et al., 2018; Morina et al., 2018).

Somatization (SSD in *DSM-5*), although potentially arising from a variety of factors, has been linked on multiple occasions to a history of childhood maltreatment, especially sexual abuse (e.g., Iloson et al., 2021; Springs & Friedrich, 1992), as well as other traumatic events, such as war, disaster, or adult assault (Beckham et al., 1998; Kimerling & Calhoun, 1994). The reason for this association is unclear, although possibilities include (a) the effects of sustained autonomic arousal on organ systems especially responsive to sympathetic activation and (b) posttraumatic perceptions of vulnerability (with subsequent hypervigilance) based on where in the body the trauma was most salient (e.g., chronic pelvic pain in sexual abuse survivors; Briere, 1992).

Somatic symptoms also may represent *idioms of distress* (American Psychiatric Association, 2022; Nichter, 1981) in some cultures, such that physical symptoms function as ways to express nonphysical concerns. As a result, culture-bound somatic syndromes have been described in several studies (e.g., L. J. Moore et al., 2001). Kirmayer (1996) noted the following:

> This idiomatic use of symptoms allows people to draw attention to and metaphorically comment on the nature of their quandaries. When reduced to symptoms of a disorder [by clinicians], this meaningful personal and social dimension of distress may be lost. . . . In this regard, as with conversion

responses, somatic symptoms may allow communication of posttraumatic distress and symptomatology within cultures where psychological symptoms are either unacceptable or not easily expressed. (p. 133)

Functional Neurological Symptom Disorder

To meet diagnostic criteria for functional neurological symptom disorder (FNSD; also referred to as *conversion disorder*), the individual must have "[o]ne or more symptoms of altered voluntary motor or sensory function" with "evidence of incompatibility between the symptom and recognized neurological or medical conditions" (American Psychiatric Association, 2022, p. 360). Typical FNSD symptoms include paralysis, loss of ability to speak (aphonia), abnormal movements, blindness, deafness, weakness, difficulties swallowing, "stocking-glove" anesthesia, and seizures. Conversion disorder was initially linked to guilt and conflict in the early psychoanalytic literature (Akagi & House, 2002). However, most empirically based analyses suggest an association between FNSD and stress and trauma factors (American Psychiatric Association, 2013). Traumas frequently implicated in the clinical literature include child abuse (e.g., Hailes et al., 2019), combat (e.g., van der Hart et al., 2001), and torture (e.g., Van Ommeren et al., 2001).

CULTURE-BOUND TRAUMA RESPONSES

As indicated at the beginning of this chapter, posttraumatic presentations are influenced by a variety of individual, environmental, and sociocultural variables. People from different cultures often experience trauma and express posttraumatic distress in ways that diverge from what is found in Anglo-European societies (Hinton et al., 2013; Kirmayer et al., 2010). As Marsella and colleagues (1996) noted, individuals from non-European cultures "often fail to meet PTSD diagnostic criteria because they lack avoidant/numbing symptoms despite the presence of reexperiencing and arousal symptoms" (p. 533). Furthermore, in some cultures, classic PTSD symptoms involve more somatic and dissociative symptoms than are found in North American groups (Marsella et al., 1996).

Although these symptoms may be considered culture-bound stress responses (Yamada & Marsella, 2013) or *cultural concepts of distress* (American Psychiatric Association, 2022, p. 871), PTSD itself should also be considered at least partially culture bound, because it best describes the posttraumatic symptoms of those raised in Anglo-European countries (Alford, 2016; Marsella, 2010). The "Cultural Concepts of Distress" section of the *DSM-5-TR* lists examples of several culture-specific syndromes that are potentially trauma related, including the following (American Psychiatric Association, 2022, pp. 874–878):

- *ataque de nervios* ("attack of nerves"),
- *nervios* ("nerves"),
- *khyâl* ("wind," attacks that involve symptoms similar to panic attacks),
- *kufungisisa* ("thinking too much," as a sign of distress, similar to excessive worry or rumination), and
- *susto* ("fright," when a frightening event causes the soul to leave the body, resulting in a range of distressing symptoms).

Notably, the *DSM-5-TR* specifically allows the coding of culture-bound stress disorders under the rubric of other specified trauma- and stressor-related disorders. This cultural variation does not mean that individuals from other societies or cultures do not ever develop PTSD; PTSD symptoms are commonly reported by traumatized people to some extent regardless of culture or geographic locale (e.g., J. P. Wilson & Tang, 2007).

CONCLUSION

This chapter outlined a number of disorders that are either intrinsically associated with traumatic events or that may arise from traumatic events or processes. It also identified several stress-related syndromes that, although not often seen in mainstream North American or European society, are prevalent in other cultures. As the role of trauma in psychological disorders becomes more widely understood by practitioners and researchers, other diagnoses probably will be found to relate, in some instances, to traumatic stress as well. Trauma can be etiologically associated with mental disorders in at least two different ways: first, by directly producing posttraumatic responses (e.g., as in PTSD, ASD, or the dissociative disorders); and second, by triggering an already latent or prepotent process into a visible disorder (e.g., acute exacerbations of chronic schizophrenia or depression, secondary to a major stressor).

It is likely that as psychological diagnosis becomes more sophisticated, clinicians will find that the very notion of dichotomously present-or-absent disorders is an oversimplification. Especially with regard to PTSD-related phenomena, it is probably more accurate to refer to posttraumatic spectrum responses of various types that—if determined to be of sufficient severity or frequency—may meet diagnostic criteria and become a disorder.

Fortunately, although the exact etiologic pathway to various diagnoses may not be fully known and the longstanding controversy between symptom continua and discrete disorders has yet to be settled, the clinician need not resolve these issues in order to assess potentially posttraumatic states. As we will discuss in later chapters, the examiner's responsibility is to evaluate the current level and configuration of symptomatology presented by the client, to determine whether their self-reported (or otherwise determined) history appears to contain traumatic events sufficient to produce such symptoms, to consider the relative contribution of mediating risk factors, and to make, if necessary, hypotheses about potential links between these two phenomena. Although a clearly appropriate *DSM-5-TR* diagnosis may arise from this process, in some cases it will not; the symptomatology—although potentially of clinical import—may be too diverse or of insufficient intensity or frequency to justify a specific *DSM* label. In many cases, the examiner will also not be able to state with absolute certainty that a given disorder or symptom pattern arose directly and exclusively from a specific traumatic event, as discussed in the next chapter.

Nevertheless, posttraumatic states are relatively common; they often arise from events that trigger clinical, judicial, or compensatory interventions from society (and thus require detailed evaluation), yet they may be overlooked by the clinical evaluator who has insufficient information on posttraumatic responses. The remainder of this book addresses the various issues that must be considered if an accurate and meaningful psychological assessment is to be made.

PART **II** GENERAL ISSUES IN
THE ASSESSMENT
OF POSTTRAUMATIC
STRESS

3 CRITICAL ISSUES IN TRAUMA-RELEVANT ASSESSMENT

Psychological assessment of posttraumatic states, whether by diagnostic interview or psychometric testing, must take into account certain issues if it is to be successful. Among these are the quality of the evaluation environment, the need to assess both trauma-related and more generic symptoms, the potential for the client to under- or overreport traumatic events and symptoms, the effects of assessor interactional style on client test data, and the limits of evaluator testimony in the courtroom. This chapter discusses each of these, along with the advantages and disadvantages of racial and ethnic normative adjustments, issues associated with interpreting test results with nonheterotypic clients, and the complexities associated with using tests translated and normed on one population (typically U.S. residents) with clients from other countries and cultures.

APPROACH TO ASSESSMENT

Because trauma victims, by definition, have been exposed to danger and intrusion, it is not uncommon for them to approach the assessment process with trepidation, if not distrust. When the trauma has recently occurred or

https://doi.org/10.1037/0000452-003
Psychological Assessment of Adult Posttraumatic States: Phenomenology, Diagnosis, and Measurement, Third Edition, by E. M. Eadie and J. Briere

is especially overwhelming in some way, the victim may experience psychological evaluation as yet another component of the traumatic event itself and may view the evaluator as an additional stressor. For example, crisis workers occasionally find that their attempts to engage in initial mental status evaluations and triage with victims of mass trauma are perceived by some victims as intrusive, bureaucratic, or even malignant.

In fact, the assessment process may be inherently stressful for some (Litz et al., 1992). The request that a survivor describe (and thereby recall) traumatic events can reactivate upsetting memories and painful affects, producing more posttraumatic stress than may have been present before the interview. For example, victims of political torture may sharply fear what they view as interrogation by an authority figure; adult survivors of childhood abuse may expect betrayal or violation rather than assistance; and rape victims may experience renewed distress if evaluated by someone in some way similar (e.g., by gender, ethnicity, or personal characteristics) to the rapist.

In some sense, the assessor is constrained by a psychological version of the uncertainty principle. Just as observation of an event in physics inevitably changes that event, aspects of the assessment process may temporarily alter the client's current state and influence the results of assessment. A classic example of how this dynamic can go awry is in some forensic or clinical evaluations where the examiner appears unnecessarily distant and skeptical, is excessively abrupt or intrusive with questions, or is, ironically, too invasively sympathetic regarding the assumed traumatic experience. In response, the interviewee may become avoidant (e.g., nondisclosing or dissociative) or restimulated (e.g., angry or cognitively disorganized), ultimately leading to an inaccurate psychological report regarding their history or current psychological symptoms.

The evaluator should take this reactive dimension of trauma assessment into account, so that the client is not unduly stressed by the interview and the resulting assessment data are not contaminated by the client's negative reactions to assessment or the assessor. In some instances, this approach may mean that certain psychological tests (e.g., projective instruments) are not administered until the client is more stable and less distressed; in other cases, even a trauma-based mental status examination or detailed description of the traumatic event may have to be delayed. Despite the sometimes pressing need to acquire assessment data from the client, the ultimate issue is the client's continuing well-being and the importance of avoiding any further harm.

For these reasons, the assessing clinician should work to provide a manifestly safe evaluation environment and to develop as much rapport with the client as possible. Among other things, this approach requires that the evaluator

- be sensitive to the client's current situation, stressors, and level of functioning;
- pace the interview so that the client is not overwhelmed by questions or demands for information;
- explain testing procedures in advance; and
- obtain the client's implicit, if not explicit, permission for each step in the assessment process.

More generally, the clinician must attempt to find a psychological place in relation to the trauma survivor that is neither so distant as to be nonempathic or uncaring nor so close as to be intrusive or threatening.

It is also generally a good idea to inform the client beforehand that assessment may be somewhat stressful—without, of course, suggesting that it is intrinsically injurious. In this way, the client is more able to give informed consent and is, to some extent, prepared for possible assessment-related distress. In some cases, the examiner may even debrief the client after the evaluation, inviting them to discuss, process, and place into context the impacts of talking about the trauma.

Interestingly, however, even a brief discussion (written or otherwise) of traumatic events has been shown to significantly decrease psychological symptoms and increase indices of physical health (e.g., E. J. Brown & Heimberg, 2001; Pennebaker, 2018; Sloan & Marx, 2019). As well, Brabin and Berah (1995) reported that the minority of research participants in their study who found trauma questions stressful also described positive impacts of such inquiry. Thus, the potentially stressful effects of trauma-focused assessment should not be seen as necessarily enduring and may be psychologically helpful in the longer term, especially if conducted in a thoughtful and compassionate manner.

Nevertheless, on relatively rare occasions, the severely traumatized client may react adversely to the assessment process. This adverse reaction may occur either (a) because assessment stimuli (e.g., test materials or the examiner's physical or psychological characteristics) reactivate significant posttraumatic stress in an otherwise seemingly stable individual or (b) because, especially in acute trauma settings, the client is already sufficiently destabilized that any additional psychic demands exacerbate their posttraumatic state. In either instance, the evaluatee may present with evidence of increased stress, such as panic, anger, flashbacks, dissociative responses, or even tangentiality or confusion.

Obviously, in such unusual cases, further assessment is almost always contraindicated, and the primary task becomes emotional stabilization. Clinical experience suggests that this process may be aided by reduced stimulation, reassurance, and grounding. First, the evaluator typically terminates the assessment process as soon as is reasonably possible, generally refrains from further activating inquiries or statements, and reduces environmental stimuli that could cue or trigger posttraumatic stress. If evaluation took place near the traumatic event (e.g., near a disaster site or in an emergency setting where other victims are visible), the clinician may consider moving the non-injured client to a less stimulating environment. If the upset is caused by a testing stimulus or items on a psychological inventory, the examiner may choose to visibly put away such materials, so that direct restimulation will be reduced and symbolic termination of the upsetting event may occur.

Reassurance and grounding are also important parts of deescalating evaluation-related distress or disturbance. The client is typically reminded of the safety of the assessment environment, and their emotional reactions are framed as reasonable given their situation. During this normalization process, the evaluator's voice and demeanor should be calming and reassuring. When necessary, the clinician may draw the client's attention to the concrete aspects of the immediate environment in such a way as to distract from escalating internal states. When the client has returned to a more stable emotional state, assessment may be either carefully reinitiated or delayed to a later point in time.

Goals of Trauma-Relevant Assessment

Assuming that assessment can occur without overstressing the client, a central issue concerns the actual goal of such evaluation. For example, in the assessment of a rape victim, is the ultimate intent to determine (a) whether the victim's current symptoms are directly attributable to the rape; (b) whether the victim is experiencing posttraumatic distress or disorder; or (c) the extent to which the victim is suffering from any sort of psychological disturbance, including posttraumatic stress?

Although the first option might seem important, it is often the case that a given psychological presentation cannot be absolutely linked to an earlier traumatic event. Even if the client reports definitive symptoms of acute stress disorder (ASD) or acute posttraumatic stress disorder (PTSD), it is possible that some other traumatic experience produced some or all of the symptoms in question. Even more problematic are chronic PTSD, dissociative, and personality-level symptoms, because the etiology of these responses may reside far in the past. In instances in which a cause-and-effect relationship must be specifically evaluated (e.g., in some forensic situations), important issues include the temporal sequence (e.g., Did the posttraumatic disturbance appear after the traumatic event, in the absence of other intervening traumas?) and the nature of the intrusive symptoms (e.g., Does the client report flashbacks or intrusive images and memories of the specific rape experience in question?). If these two conditions are met and the validity of the test data can be assured, the clinician may be able to hypothesize (but not guarantee) that the rape, in fact, produced the client's posttraumatic symptoms.

More typically, the traumatic event may be long past (e.g., in childhood or at some point earlier in life), the symptoms may be less clear-cut (e.g., dissociative symptoms or depression), and other negative life events may have intervened between the hypothesized stressor and the observed clinical state. It may also be the case that other traumas or victimization experiences occurred prior to the identified stressor and the specific linkages between one traumatic event or another and the resulting symptoms are difficult, or impossible, to disentangle. In such cases, and in the absence of other relevant data, the evaluating clinician may be left with the conclusion that (a) the client's report of an earlier trauma(s) appears to be valid, and (b) their current state is consistent with the possibility that the trauma produced the current symptom pattern, but that (c) a definitive connection between these two events cannot be asserted absolutely. In other words, there is rarely a psychological litmus test for the existence or effects of a given trauma, especially one long past. Fortunately, other than in some forensic contexts (e.g., civil litigation for psychological damages), this trauma–response connection need not be definitive. Instead, the clinician may determine that the best-fitting hypothesis is that the trauma and the posttraumatic stress are related, without ruling out other potential etiologies.

The second issue, that of determining whether a posttraumatic condition exists, is typically possible in a sensitive and competent psychological evaluation. In certain instances, however, even this goal may be elusive. As noted in Chapter 6, many generic psychological tests are relatively insensitive to posttraumatic states, and they instead misclassify such symptoms as evidence of other disorders, such as a personality disorder or psychosis. As well, the clinician unfamiliar with (or negatively predisposed toward) posttraumatic disturbance may misinterpret or overlook existing trauma-related symptoms in a clinical interview. Finally, as discussed later in this chapter, the client's need for avoidance may cause them to deny or mask posttraumatic symptomatology, thereby reducing the visibility of such symptoms during evaluation. Given these issues, the most effective evaluator will be familiar with the complexities of posttraumatic clinical presentation, will administer trauma-sensitive psychological tests along with a sensitive clinical interview (see Chapters 5 and 7), and will work to provide an evaluation environment that minimizes the presence of client avoidance or distortion.

Even though the assessment focus may be on posttraumatic stress and stressors, the ultimate goal of a competent evaluation is not solely to define the relationship between aversive experiences and outcomes or to identify specific posttraumatic difficulties. Instead, the client's entire symptom experience should be assessed. For example, although an earthquake victim's ASD is an obvious target for evaluation, their preexisting obsessive-compulsive symptoms and current panic disorder are also important components of the clinical picture. Similarly, individuals with psychotic disorders or certain personality traits or disorders are thought to be especially prone to PTSD when exposed to moderate stressors (Buswell et al., 2021); thus, a complete psychological assessment will include data on these clinical antecedents as well. Finally, some nontrauma-related symptoms (e.g., certain obsessional, psychotic, or anxiety symptoms) may mimic posttraumatic symptomatology. In such instances, failure to consider all relevant diagnostic possibilities may lead to a misidentification of posttraumatic disturbance.

Generally, as noted in Chapter 2, diagnostic notions such as complex PTSD or posttraumatic depression reflect the fact that posttraumatic stress is often present in the context of other symptoms and disorders. Studies suggest, for example, that those with PTSD may also suffer from other, coexisting disorders such as depression, anxiety disorders (especially panic disorder, phobias, and obsessive-compulsive disorder), alcohol and drug abuse, and borderline or antisocial personality disorder (Breslau & Davis, 1992; Qassem et al., 2021). This overlap appears to represent not only the comorbidity of various disorders with PTSD but also the fact that some PTSD symptoms are similar to those for depressive and anxiety disorders (e.g., Flory & Yehuda, 2015; Kessler et al., 1995). Such symptom and disorder overlap emphasizes the need to evaluate the full range of psychological disorders when assessing the traumatized client.

In summary, clinical evaluation of trauma victims must take into account clients' entire psychological experience, including the complexity of potentially etiologic, predisposing, and moderating events, and the possibility of significant comorbidity with other, less trauma-related conditions. Failure to consider these broader issues may result in erroneous conclusions or unnecessarily constrained clinical data.

AVOIDANCE AND UNDERREPORTING

It is not surprising that traumatic events can motivate the development and use of avoidance strategies. Avoidance may present as emotional or cognitive suppression, denial, dissociation, memory distortion, or involvement in activities that numb or distract (i.e., distress reduction activities). For example, a combat veteran may attempt to suppress thoughts about their war experiences, may avoid situations where they have to talk about the war, may enter a dissociative state when exposed to combat-relevant stimuli, or may use alcohol or drugs to numb posttraumatic distress.

Although such avoidance strategies can be superficially adaptive, they can easily interfere with accurate psychological evaluation. Regarding the latter, the client's tendency to avoid or attenuate distress may alter their response to psychological assessment, in some instances leading to a significant under-reporting of a trauma history or posttraumatic effects. This underreporting may especially occur if a given assessment requires the victim to recall or reexperience trauma-related events. More generally, R. S. Epstein (1993) noted that the "avoidant symptoms of PTSD can serve as a 'self-cloaking' device that may hinder or prevent timely diagnosis" (p. 457).

Avoidance also may present in the form of *psychogenic amnesia*, in which case the victim may have insufficient recall of traumatic experiences and thus will not report them during the evaluation interview. As noted in Chapter 2, several studies (e.g., Elliott & Briere, 1995; G. S. Goodman et al., 2003) suggest that some instances of childhood or adult trauma may be relatively unavailable to conscious memory for extended periods of time, during which, presumably, the subjects of these studies would deny or underestimate historical events that did, in fact, occur. Some research suggests a neurological basis for such cognitive avoidance. Anderson et al. (2004) used functional magnetic resonance imaging to demonstrate that increased prefrontal activation and reduced hippocampus activation were associated with the unconscious suppression of unwanted memories in the laboratory. By definition, such memory suppression might easily alter the trauma disclosure process.

Defensive avoidance of painful material also may suppress clients' scores on symptom measures. In a still-influential article, Shedler and colleagues (1993) demonstrated in a more general context that "standard mental health scales appear unable to distinguish between genuine mental health and the facade or illusion of mental health created by psychological defenses" (p. 1117). In support of this notion, Elliott and Briere (1994) reported on a subsample of children for whom there was compelling evidence of sexual abuse (e.g., unambiguous medical findings, photographs taken by the abuser, or abuser confession) but who nonetheless both (a) denied that they had been abused and (b) scored significantly lower than the control group (children without known sexual abuse histories) on the Trauma Symptom Checklist for Children (Briere, 1996). As Elliott and Briere (1994) noted, it is likely that these children were using denial and other cognitive avoidance strategies to keep from confronting both their abuse and its psychological effects. In the absence of outside corroboration, these children probably would have been judged as nonabused and nondistressed on interview or by psychological evaluation.

Symptom underreporting, while potentially an important issue in the assessment of abuse survivors and other traumatized individuals, is difficult to identify through psychological tests. At present, the practitioner is limited to reliance on validity scales that index defensiveness or fake-good responses. Examples include the L and K scales of the Minnesota Multiphasic Personality Inventory–3 (MMPI-3; Ben-Porath & Tellegen, 2020), the Positive Impression Management scale of the Personality Assessment Inventory (PAI; Morey, 1991, 2007), the Disclosure and Desirability indices of the Millon Clinical Multiaxial Inventory–IV (MCMI-IV; Millon et al., 2015), and the Response Level scale of the Trauma Symptom Inventory–2 (TSI-2; Briere, 2011). Unfortunately, although these validity indicators identify more extreme cases of underreporting, it is likely that many other instances will go unidentified unless the clinician can somehow detect it during the evaluation interview.

Implications for Assessment Practice

As a result of the various processes just described, the clinician should not rule out the possibility of an unreported traumatic event or trauma-related disturbance in a given individual's life history, whether the missing information occurs as a result of conscious suppression of upsetting material or more unconscious defensive processes. Importantly, however, the possibility of significant avoidance-based underreporting does not mean that an individual who is symptomatic but denies a victimization history, or who reports a trauma but denies symptomatology, is necessarily in denial about a specific traumatic event or suppressing expression of posttraumatic stress. Furthermore, although complete dissociation of trauma-related memories or complete denial of symptoms in a symptomatic person is possible, such responses are not the norm and should not be automatically assumed unless there are specific data in support of that hypothesis.

Ultimately, the best approach to situations in which trauma and/or traumatic distress are denied but the clinician suspects there are some contradictory data is to

- avoid making assumptions either way regarding potential underreporting,
- examine any psychometric data that bear on the issues of potential underreporting, and
- provide the conditions under which the client hopefully has less need to avoid or deny trauma-related difficulties during the assessment process.

For example, a combat veteran presents with a significant trauma history and yet denies any symptoms of PTSD, despite exhibiting obvious signs of both emotional numbing and autonomic hyperarousal. Although the veteran may be suppressing or avoiding combat-related posttraumatic stress, it is also possible that another comorbidity (e.g., extreme anxiety or depression) is the primary generator of their current symptoms, or another adverse event (e.g., childhood abuse) may be more etiological. In this context, the clinician may be most effective to the extent that they avoid arguing about or challenging the client's narrative, and instead validate the client's ongoing experience and provide safety and nonjudgement during the assessment session, including not pressuring the client to disclose things that are currently too upsetting to acknowledge or that are not, in fact, relevant to their current psychological state. Apropos of this general approach, it is not unusual for a previously avoidant client to become more forthcoming about their history and its effects as the therapeutic relationship grows and the client internalizes the therapist's supportive stance (Briere & Lanktree, 2012).

Actual client avoidance and nondisclosure, however, may not yield to the assessor's best efforts. When this occurs, it is important that the clinician not definitively state in any report that the client is falsely denying or repressing a trauma or its effects. Instead, the best approach is typically (a) to note the presence of symptoms based on psychological testing, if they are present; (b) to describe the results of psychometric validity testing, including whether any underreporting scales are elevated; and (c) in obvious cases, to note intrainterview signs of avoidance (e.g., numbing, sudden dissociative reactions, or hyper- or nonresponse to trauma-related questions); and then (d) to discuss relevant possibilities—including potential underreporting—that account for the test and interview data. We recommend that this discussion not include any definitive statements about whether a given trauma did or did not occur, or whether, in the absence of other information, the client is underreporting or accurately disclosing symptomatology.

OVERREPORTING

In contrast to underreporting, some proportion of individuals may overreport or misrepresent trauma histories or trauma-related symptoms. In some cases, inaccurate reporting may represent a conscious or unconscious cry for help by individuals seeking attention to injuries or suffering that they fear otherwise would be overlooked. There may be financial influences as well: In most Western cultures, victims can file suit against their alleged perpetrators, and some institutions (e.g., the U.S. Department of Veterans Affairs and state victim compensation boards) appropriately provide financial support or compensation to those who have been traumatized.

Occasionally, overreporting of trauma histories or symptoms may occur in the context of psychosis or severe personality disorders. Yet borderline personality disorder itself may arise from child maltreatment (among other things; as noted in Chapter 2), and recent research implicates the role of trauma in some psychotic presentations. In addition, there are no data to suggest that more disturbed individuals have a lower probability of being traumatized than other people, and there is considerable cause to expect that psychologically impaired or incapacitated people are easier prey for predatory individuals. As a result, the trauma or symptom reports of psychotic or personality-disordered individuals should not be discounted automatically; rather, they should be evaluated for their credibility and meaning in the same manner as any other historical statements might be considered.

In other cases, there may be concerns that the client is suffering from a factitious disorder, wherein they are driven to overreport traumas or symptoms as a result of psychological disturbance. Although factition is often associated with attempts to appear as if one has a physical disorder or injury, most trauma specialists encounter individuals whose presenting description of traumatic events and posttraumatic stress appears to serve a need for psychological, medical, or other attention (Lacoursiere, 1993). For example, an individual without military experience may present to a crisis center or outpatient clinic with credible reports of combat trauma and resultant posttraumatic stress. Although factitious trauma presentations are relatively uncommon in clinical populations, they are not unheard of and should be considered in instances in which the presenting problem seems overstated, contradicted by other information, or in some other way suspect.

Finally, concerns about rampant "false memories" of childhood abuse, especially raised in the 1990s and early 2000s (e.g., McHugh, 2008), suggest the possibility that some clinicians might encourage the production of pseudomemories of abuse in susceptible clients, referred to as *false memory syndrome* (Olio, 2004). These concerns appear to have been overstated in previous years and were primarily raised as a legal defense by individuals accused of abusing their children (Dalenberg et al., 2020), and they have not been validated as an actual syndrome or disorder in any diagnostic system (Rix, 2000). However, it is likely that some instances of pseudomemory production do, in fact, occur, and they can have potentially devastating consequences for innocent parties, in addition to complicating the psychological assessment process (Lindsay & Briere, 1997). As Courtois (1995) noted, while referencing J. L. Herman (1992b):

> [T]he therapist must be technically neutral while being cognizant of the prevalence and possibility of an abuse history. But technical neutrality does not mean

avoidance of asking the appropriate questions and cognizance does not mean that the therapist assumes sexual abuse to the exclusion of other issues. The therapist should be open to the possibility of other childhood events and trauma that might account for the symptom picture and should not prematurely foreclose these other possibilities. (p. 21)

As with underreporting, it is somewhat difficult to reliably identify cases of overreporting through the use of psychological tests. In some cases, overreporting may be detected through validity scale scores, such as elevations on the following: the Infrequency-Psychopathology (Fp) scale, Dissimulation (Ds) scale, and F-K index of the MMPI-2, MMPI-2-RF, and MMPI-3; the Negative Impression Management (NIM) scale of the PAI (Morey, 1991, 2007); the Debasement (Z) scale of the MCMI-IV (Millon et al., 2015); the Atypical Response (ATR) scale of the TSI-2 (Briere, 2011); and the Structured Interview of Reported Symptoms–2 (SIRS-2; Rogers et al., 2010). However, individuals who have experienced interpersonal victimization, combat, or other severe traumas tend to score more deviantly on such validity scales, thereby lessening to some degree their usefulness with trauma survivors (Elhai et al., 2002; Frueh et al., 2000; Hyer et al., 1987). For example, the elevated invalidity scores of some Vietnam combat veterans and child abuse survivors appear to reflect the chronic posttraumatic stress, dissociation, cognitive distortions, affective symptoms, or substance abuse often found in these groups, as opposed to motivated symptom overendorsement (e.g., Jordan et al., 1992; Klotz Flitter et al., 2003; D. W. Smith & Frueh, 1996). Given this confounding of validity responses with posttraumatic symptomatology, the clinician or forensic evaluator is faced with a difficult tradeoff: Does one strictly apply validity cutoffs, thereby catching some cases of overreporting but also potentially eliminating valid protocols of especially traumatized individuals? Or does one use more liberal cutoffs to retain valid trauma protocols, yet run the risk of incorrectly interpreting overreported or false test responses as valid?

In some cases, the clinician may choose to avoid using certain validity indicators or scales entirely, because their item content overlaps with valid trauma-related symptoms or concerns. For example, the NIM scale includes items about having multiple personalities, having amnesia, and not having positive memories from childhood (Stadnik et al., 2013). In addition, the SIRS-2, by virtue of item overlap, can overclassify people with complex posttraumatic outcomes, including dissociative identity disorder, as feigning (Brand et al., 2006).

Implications for Assessment Practice

Given the reliable correlation between trauma and later psychological difficulties, it is recommended that clinicians inquire about childhood and adult traumas as a routine part of all clinical evaluations in which such questions can be tolerated and are likely to be valid. These questions should be posed as a regular part of history-taking, as opposed to being given special attention or emphasis in such a way as to suggest that a specific answer is desired (for more on gathering a trauma history, see Chapter 4). We advise clinicians to avoid such biased questioning, especially during hypnosis, drug-assisted interviews, or within any other context that might capitalize on suggestibility or lead the client to report more than they actually recall.

Thus, a competent forensic assessment during a psychological damages lawsuit, for example, should consider the possibility of malingering (R. I. Simon, 2003). Similarly, a more treatment-focused evaluation should not overlook the possibility of intentional misrepresentation, because such phenomena obviously require different sorts of intervention strategies. This possibility should be a normal rule-out issue, however. Clinical experience suggests that false reports of trauma or trauma-related symptomatology are rarer in nonforensic clinical settings and should not be automatically assumed, just as other reports should not be automatically accepted in their entirety.

In this context, validity scales that evaluate symptom overreporting can be quite useful, although they sometimes may overidentify factitious or fake-bad responding (Franklin, Repasky, et al., 2002; Frueh et al., 2000). Other scales, such as the TSI-2, may be less prone to misidentifying overreporting; instead, they may underestimate some cases of malingering, at least in analogue studies (for review, see Ales & Erdodi, 2022). Just as symptom scales should be scrutinized for their psychometric validity vis-à-vis trauma and its effects, validity scales that proport to identify overresponding should be evaluated for their accuracy and utility especially among trauma survivors.

MISIDENTIFICATION AND DISTORTION EFFECTS

Because most standard psychological tests (e.g., the MMPI or the Rorschach) were not developed at a time when psychological trauma was well recognized, these instruments may underidentify or distort trauma effects. Older instruments (see Chapter 6) may inadvertently confuse intrusive posttraumatic symptomatology with hallucinations, obsessions, primary process, or fake-bad responses; may misinterpret dissociative avoidance as fragmented thinking, chaotic internal states, or symptoms of schizophrenia; and may misidentify trauma-based cognitive phenomena (e.g., hypervigilance or generalized distrust) as evidence of paranoia or other delusional processes. Furthermore, these tests may misinterpret the effects of childhood trauma as personality disorders to the extent that they involve interpersonal difficulties, chaotic internal states, and distress reduction or other emotional avoidance activities.

This tendency for traditional measures to misinterpret posttraumatic symptoms might seemingly preclude their use in trauma assessment. However, the issue may be less that of intrinsically bad data (i.e., the test items themselves) than of erroneous interpretation (i.e., how the items and scales are understood). For example, although many sexual abuse survivors have elevations on scales 4 and 8 of the MMPI-2 (to note, the MMPI-3 no longer uses point profiles), it is often inappropriate to view these individuals as potentially schizophrenic (scale 8), psychopathic (scale 4), or borderline (e.g., a 4-8 profile; discussed in Chapter 6). Instead, examination of specific items and available subscale scores may indicate the presence of nonpsychotic reexperiencing symptoms, interpersonal distrust or social alienation, and dissociative responses, as well as accurate reporting of familial discord during childhood. Thus, to the extent that more trauma-relevant interpretations can be made, standard psychological tests can be a helpful part of the trauma assessment process. This is important because there are tremendous databases available on individuals' responses to the MMPI and its later editions and to the Millon inventories, Rorschach, and other tests—data that can be well used when applied with care.

Important issues to consider when using traditional psychological test data are at least fourfold. First, the test itself must be generally understood, in terms of how it was developed and normed; its relevant psychometric qualities, including its reliability, sensitivity (the percentage of instances that it detects actual cases of the disorder in question), and specificity (the percentage of instances that it correctly detects noncases of the disorder); and the underlying theory on which interpretation of scores is based. For example, a test normed on a relatively homogeneous sample of Midwestern adults may have diminished applicability to an African American combat veteran with severe and chronic PTSD. Similarly, a projective test interpretation system that regularly relies on traditional psychoanalytic theory may be of limited validity in the assessment of an individual who was repeatedly assaulted by a family member as a child.

Second, the item domain of the instrument should be evaluated: Do the items tap the labeled construct well, or can they misinterpret other phenomena as evidence of the construct? To the extent that the items within a given scale reflect multiple phenomena, some of which are more trauma relevant than others, are there interpretable subscales available (e.g., on the PAI)? Because such subscales are typically more unidimensional than summary scale scores, their meaning with regard to the client's current state may be more transparent and therefore more helpful.

Third, the presence of more specific trauma scales within the instrument should be taken into account. The MMPI-2, PAI, and MCMI-IV, for example, each have PTSD scales, whereas the MMPI-3 only has the more general Anxiety-Related Experiences scale (see Chapter 6). Although the PTSD scales on the PAI, MCMI-IV, and MMPI-2 have less than perfect content coverage (i.e., all underestimate certain posttraumatic symptoms and some contain less trauma-relevant symptoms such as depression; described in Chapter 6), they may alert the examiner to the possibility of significant posttraumatic stress and thus to alternate explanations for other scale elevations. Furthermore, ad hoc, trauma-specific scoring rules for a given instrument often are available, such as the Traumatic Content Index (Armstrong & Loewenstein, 1990) for the Rorschach, thereby adding more information for interpretation.

Fourth, standardized, more generic psychological tests should be augmented with additional, more trauma-specific instruments. Because the notion of posttraumatic stress is relatively new, however, there are a limited (albeit growing) number of standardized instruments available in this area thus far. Trauma-focused tests (a) should be normed on large, sociodemographically diverse samples; (b) should have demonstrated reliability and validity; and (c) should measure a number of areas of posttraumatic disturbance. Regarding the latter, a scale that yields a single summary PTSD score is often less helpful because PTSD involves four separate, only moderately correlated components—reexperiencing, avoidance, numbing and negative cognitions and mood, and hyperarousal (Chapter 2)—each of which may vary in magnitude in any specific instance. The most useful measures provide scores on each component, so that a more detailed assessment of posttraumatic stress can be made. For example, whereas a summary measure of PTSD (e.g., as found in the R scale of the MCMI-III and MCMI-IV) might indicate that an assault victim is experiencing moderately high posttraumatic stress, a more detailed instrument might suggest that their levels of intrusion and arousal are high but their avoidance is within normal limits.

ISSUES ASSOCIATED WITH NORMATIVE GROUPS

A key characteristic of standardized tests is their use of a normative dataset, allowing comparison of a given person's test responses to those of a representative sample of the general population. On clinical tests, client endorsements that are significantly greater than the relevant normative group scores are usually interpreted as evidence of psychological disturbance or symptomatology. The role of norms in standardized testing is sufficiently important that modern test guidelines generally mandate their use whenever possible in assessment practice (American Educational Research Association et al., 2014). Yet the validity of normative comparisons is limited by the actual representativeness and appropriateness of the normative sample. Norms may be misleading to the extent that they do not include people with the full and representative range of critical demographic characteristics such as age, sex, race and ethnicity, income, gender identity, and geographic location (American Educational Research Association et al., 2014).

In most cases, it is important that the normative sample be relatively large and that the proportions of important demographics match relevant census data. Doing so ensures, for example, that a middle-aged African American woman's scores on a given trauma test can be compared to a group that includes those with similar individual and intersecting characteristics. Although this is obviously a good start, it is likely insufficient in some cases. It may not be enough to compare an 18-year-old's scores on an externalizing measure to a normative group that includes *some* young adults; it may also be important to compare their scores *only* to other young adults. In this way, for example, the more frequent sexual behavior of a younger person might not be considered as extreme as might be the case if the normative group included a significant number of older people who were less sexually active.

Yet there can be problems with normative subgroup comparisons, especially for race and gender. Perhaps most importantly, comparing client scores to others with the same demographics may underidentify symptomatology and may confound demographic status with social inequality. For example, if a demographic group (e.g., people of color) is known to have a greater likelihood of marginalization, trauma exposure, and posttraumatic difficulties, the client's score will have to be especially elevated in order to appear clinically significant relative to others with similar demographic risk factors and therefore potentially similar symptomatology. In other words, racial and ethnic or gender norms may underestimate psychological problems or symptoms when the reference group is composed of others who also suffer.

Furthermore, some demographic categories (e.g., race) are complex and may not even represent meaningful biological constructs (American Psychological Association, 2019). When comparing the scores of a person to other people of the "same" race, the issue arises: Are all people identified as Black, for example, culturally or geographically equivalent, such that their scores can be directly compared? Or should one only compare the scores of a Black person from the Caribbean (e.g., Jamaica or Haiti) to other Black Caribbean individuals, as opposed to Black people whose ancestors are directly from Africa or another place? In light of such complexities, as well as the dangers associated with potentially underestimating symptoms when the comparison group has been exposed to multiple adversities, we, like others (e.g., Gasquoine, 2009), recommend that racial or ethnic norms not be employed when interpreting psychological tests, perhaps especially those investigating trauma. Fortunately, race-based norms are the exception for most trauma-relevant tests (e.g., as opposed to some neuropsychological measures [American Academy of Clinical Neuropsychology, 2021]), and thus can be avoided by assessing clinicians without difficulty.

Similar exclusions might be made for using norms based on traditional binary notions of male and female. Not all people identify as either of these gender options, and those who do may not currently identify with a gender that they were assigned at birth. As a result, traditional gender norms run the risk of excluding those who do not identify themselves in binary fashion and may underrepresent potentially important differences between those identifying, for example, as cisgender as opposed to transgender. Similarly, like racial norming, there are significant gender differences in trauma exposure and posttraumatic stress, typically meaning that those who identify as female have experienced more abuse, assault, and other interpersonal adversities than those identifying as male, thereby potentially requiring higher symptom endorsement by a given woman before it can be seen as clinically elevated relative to other women.

In contrast, there are many sex and gender differences documented in the literature, such that it is not always advantageous to compare, for example, women to a normative group that also contains men. When within-sex/gender norms are used, it may be helpful (a) to consider the potentially mediating or moderating role of adverse social variables and (b) to acknowledge the potential underestimation of psychological symptomatology associated with comparing a potentially traumatized person to a normative group in which trauma is also common.

Interpreting Test Scores With Transgender and Nonbinary Clients

An only recently appreciated phenomenon involves the self-identified nonbinary or transgendered person who, in the course of their treatment or forensic evaluation, requires psychological assessment. Because they do not identify as male or female based on their biological sex or gender assigned at birth (i.e., their *cis status*), it is often unclear whether their responses should be compared with male or female normative data or with no norms at all. Although sex differences on many scales involve only a few *T*-score points, interpreting test scores of a nonbinary or a noncis-identifying person based on standard gender norms may serve to discount or contradict their current gender identity (i.e., *misgender* them) and may contribute to misleading assessment results. In other cases, if the client has just recently transitioned away from the gender they were assigned at birth, their lifetime socialization as a cisgendered male or female may mean that traditional gender norms are more relevant for interpretation of test scores. Although the field in general, and professional guidelines specifically, do not mandate a specific approach to this conundrum, a review of the literature suggests the following options:

- *Avoid sex or gender norms entirely.* In general, this means the clinician only employs measures or interviews that are not normed on sex or gender (American Psychological Association, n.d.).

- *Use tests that have specific nonbinary/noncis norms* (American Psychological Association, n.d.). Although quite rare at present, growing professional awareness of different gender identities hopefully will allow clinicians to compare, for example, a nonbinary person's test responses to a representative sample of other nonbinary people.

- *Calculate T-scores using both male and female norms, and then, in consultation with the client, choose the reference group that seems most relevant* (Keo-Meier & Fitzgerald, 2017). This option, although potentially more expensive or time-consuming because it involves repeat scoring, is growing in popularity because it lets the data inform normative choice and empowers the client to take an active role in deciding to whom they are best compared.

- *Determine which norms to use based on how long the client has lived as their current gender identity, with longer periods of time and, potentially, any hormone therapy or surgery* (Keo-Meier et al., 2015) *supporting the use of norms based on their current gender status* (Webb et al., 2016). This determination should be made by the client, not the clinician, and no official timeline can be uniformly adhered to in all cases. Instead, the client, in consultation with the clinician, must make a subjective determination about whether they have been living as a given gender for long enough to best be compared to their current gender peers or the gender they were assigned at birth.

- *Use norms associated with the client's currently identified gender* (Webb et al., 2016). This approach often not only honors the client's self-perception and wishes, but it also aligns with preliminary information that the neurobiology of transgender people is often more similar to the gender they identify with than to what was assigned at birth (Cantor, 2011).

In all cases, however, the choice of which normative group to use must ultimately reside with the client, and the clinician must be careful not to impose their own judgments or opinions when considering the appropriate normative group. Finally, whatever the decision, the assessment report should discuss the relevant issues and rationale for whatever normative group (and associated *T*-scores) was ultimately decided upon and used.

Using Tests Normed in the United States With People From Other Geographic and Linguistic Groups

Normative issues also extend more generally to geography and language. It is not uncommon, for example, for (a) English-speaking people living in other countries and (b) non-English speakers in North America and elsewhere to be administered psychological tests that employ English-speaker, U.S. population norms.

In the former case, individuals living in Canada, the United Kingdom, Australia and New Zealand, English-speaking Latin American and Caribbean countries, and elsewhere often are given the MMPI-3, PAI, MCMI-IV, TSI-2, and other popular tests that were originally developed in the United States. In cases where the cultures and demographics are broadly similar (e.g., Canada), this may not be especially problematic. However, in other instances, the client may live in a society that is more culturally disparate, where there may be considerably more (or less) adversities (e.g., wars, flagrant human rights violations) than experienced by the normative group. To the extent that the client's culture and social environment differ from the normative sample, testing may seriously conflate psychological issues with culture and trauma exposure and may be relatively insensitive to specific culture-bound symptoms and disorders.

In the case of translated but not renormed psychological tests, the situation may be even more problematic. Not only are there similar cultural issues at stake, but it is also rare that a test developed in English can be perfectly translated into another language—in fact, some English words may not even have an equivalent in another language. As a result, for example, a given item endorsement in one language relative to another may reflect not only cultural issues and different lived experiences but also inaccurate or distorted meaning as a function of the translation process. When English-language norms are applied in this scenario, misinterpretation is likely.

Because most tests, perhaps especially trauma ones, were developed in North America, there may be few choices or alternatives to at least occasional use of such measures in different geographical contexts. However, it is incumbent on the clinician to assess the fit between the client's culture and language and that of the normative sample. When the differences appear relatively minor, the test may be administered while taking any cultural, geographical, or language issues into account, and the clinician should discuss in their assessment report any concerns regarding potential limitations to any interpretations and conclusions. When the gap between the client and the normative group is large, use of English-language norms may not be possible. Instead, the evaluator may have to use a formal or informal diagnostic interview, in the client's language, to avoid normative issues.

Ideally, as psychological tests are increasingly available in other languages and are accompanied by appropriate norms, and as North American test companies increasingly offer local test norms for different countries and linguistic groups, this situation will improve. Until then, the clinician is advised to choose tests carefully, consider normative issues that might interfere with accurate interpretation, and document any variation from standardized test administration when testing non-English speakers and those from other countries and cultures.

ASSESSING SOCIAL DISCRIMINATION AND MALTREATMENT

As noted in Chapter 2, social discrimination and maltreatment (SDM), although rarely characterized as a *DSM-5-TR*–level trauma, can nevertheless result in posttraumatic stress and related psychosocial outcomes—even in the absence of life threat or physical injury (Briere et al., 2025). For this reason, a comprehensive assessment should evaluate not only the effects of classic traumatic events and other adversities but also (if relevant) the impacts of racism, sexism, anti-LGBTQ+ experiences, antisemitism, Islamophobia, and other forms of SDM (Nakamura et al., 2022). Chapter 4 describes several SDM measures, although few have been validated in clinical contexts or include all major forms of SDM. Appendix B (this volume) includes the Social Discrimination and Maltreatment Scale–Short Form (SDMS-SF; Briere, 2023; Briere et al., 2024), which briefly evaluates lifetime exposure to sexism, racism, and cis-heterosexism and can be modified to include additional types of SDM, such as antisemitism and Islamophobia. The SDMS-SF has yet to be validated in clinical environments, however, and any evaluation of SDM exposure will ideally include culturally sensitive questions about SDM in the clinical interview.

Cross-Cultural Symptoms and Disorders

As noted in Chapters 1 and 2 and elsewhere in this volume, the notion of posttraumatic stress and—to some extent—the idea of trauma itself is culturally determined. Negative events may be seen as more traumatic in one society or group than in another, by virtue of attitudes and beliefs each holds regarding the meaning of such events and their social implications for the individual exposed to them. As well, cultures vary significantly in regard to idioms of distress and underlying models they use to understand and communicate psychological injury. One culture, for example, may locate the effects of trauma in the psyche, whereas a second may assume the impact is on the body, and a third may interpret the injury as spiritual. For this reason, diagnoses such as PTSD or even depression presuppose certain etiologies, mechanisms, and phenomenologies—assumptions that may not be shared by all cultures. As a result, it is important that the clinical assessor be aware of the cultural relativity of the terms they use and the limits to their generalizability. Ultimately, the term *PTSD* may have no more value as a diagnosis than do *ataque de nervios* ("attack of nerves") or another non-*DSM/ICD* label, except as it relates to professional mental health communications about typically Western symptoms in English-speaking cultures. The implications of this are several, ranging from the realization that PTSD itself is partially a culture-bound disorder, to recognizing the need for clinicians to consider other possible forms of mental disturbance when evaluating immigrants or refugees or when engaging in outreach to traumatized people elsewhere in the world. The need for cultural awareness is obvious when one is working in a center for immigrant torture victims; it is just as significant, however, in the multicultural contexts found in most urban mental health clinics.

TRAUMA-RELATED TESTIMONY IN COURT

Although this is not a text on forensic psychology, a few points should be made with regard to expert testimony in trauma cases. There are at least two ways in which a trauma evaluator or clinician may become involved in the courts. First, the clinician who treats or evaluates trauma survivors may easily find themselves testifying with regard to one of their clients, either in a criminal case or in a civil suit. Second, a forensic evaluator may be called on to render an expert opinion regarding the presence of posttraumatic distress or disorder in someone who is involved in a criminal or civil proceeding. In our opinion, only the second clinician should offer expert testimony as to the effects of trauma and the potential validity of a specific allegation. The first clinician, to the extent that they have formed a therapeutic relationship with the client, is less likely to be objective regarding the facts of the case. Of course, this does not preclude the clinician's testimony regarding the process or content of therapy.

During testimony, the examiner would do well to adhere to four principles of expert testimony, sometimes expressed as the acronym HELP: honesty, evenhandedness, limits of expertise, and preparation (Meyers, 1996). Honesty with regard to trauma testimony typically means acknowledging an unavoidable set of realities: (a) in the absence of external corroboration, it may be impossible to determine with complete certainty whether a traumatic event has occurred; (b) it is not always possible to rule out the existence of symptom underreporting, overreporting, or malingering; and (c) when a pattern of symptoms has been established, it is rarely possible to assert with complete confidence that the symptoms in question arose entirely from a specific past traumatic event.

The fact that these limitations exist does not, however, mean that the evaluator has no role in the courtroom. First, the judge and jury may need to be appraised as to the limits of *medical certainty* with regard to potential posttraumatic states. Second, although the expert witness may not be able to provide definitive testimony regarding trauma or effect, they can assist the court in considering the various possibilities and the general likelihood of each.

In this regard, evenhandedness and an acknowledgment of the limits of expertise means that the evaluator should consider all reasonable explanations for the client's reports of trauma and posttraumatic difficulty and, to the extent that data are available, offer a carefully constrained opinion as to the likelihood of each. For example, although the interviewer may believe that, on balance, the alleged victim's reports have merit, they should also be prepared to discuss the possibility of misrepresentation or malingering. Similarly, even though an expert may have been hired by the plaintiff's attorney regarding the possibility that a given traumatic event caused short- or long-term damages, the evaluator must also consider the possibility that other antecedent or intervening negative experiences produced at least some of the symptoms in question, or that the plaintiff's reports are distorted by financial considerations. Finally, an interviewer who believes that a given allegation of posttraumatic stress is false must also consider the possibility that their expectations, demeanor, or even choice of assessment procedures precluded access to information that would have contradicted that belief. They must also accept the fact that an absence of evidence does not mean that an event did not take place. In this regard, psychological testimony that a traumatic event did not occur may be as inappropriate as unsupported testimony that it did.

Forensic experience suggests that those expert witnesses who come to significant grief in the courtroom are often those who are not well prepared regarding the actual needs of the court. Such individuals may argue one side without considering the other, failing to evaluate competing hypotheses for the complainant's allegations, symptoms, and presentation. For example, the examiner who categorically states that event A occurred and produced posttraumatic response B is less likely to be viewed as an objective expert by the judge or jury—and is much more easily discredited upon cross-examination— than the examiner who offers several potential hypotheses regarding what may have occurred. By applying relevant test and interview data to these hypotheses, along with an understanding of the relevant literature, the expert may then offer a considered but explicitly probabilistic conclusion regarding event A and posttraumatic response B. Such testimony not only honors the ethical responsibilities incumbent on psychologists, psychiatrists, and other mental health professionals, but it also carries with it greater professionalism and probity and, ultimately, greater credibility. For additional information on the forensic aspects of trauma practice, see R. I. Simon (2003) and, in the specific instance of interpersonal violence, Myers (2016).

CONCLUSION

Posttraumatic states are in some sense unique in the clinical field because of their tendency to become reactivated during the assessment of their presence. This reactivation, in turn, may distort psychological test or interview data. This concern is compounded by the fact that many evaluation approaches used in this area were developed without specific reference to posttraumatic phenomena and thus may misinterpret trauma responses as evidence of other clinical states. Because psychologists and others have only recently considered these issues in psychological assessment, no definitive information is available regarding the exact meaning of posttraumatic stress tapped by traditional assessment methodologies. As a result, some trauma survivors are likely to be seen as suffering from nontrauma-related psychopathology, and some nontraumatized individuals who seek to present themselves as posttraumatic are likely to go undetected. Thus, the examiner is on shaky ground to the extent that they absolutely conclude, based on test or interview data, that a given incident of trauma and subsequent stress have occurred and are related. Fortunately, research on the assessment and diagnosis of post-traumatic states is proceeding at a rapid pace, and new, more trauma-specific tests are being developed on an ongoing basis. The remainder of this book outlines what we have learned thus far and highlights new approaches to posttrauma assessment that substantially increase the sensitivity and specificity of trauma-relevant clinical evaluation.

4 ASSESSMENT OF TRAUMATIC EVENTS

As outlined in Chapters 1 and 2, traumatic events are not uncommon in people's lives and may lead to psychological distress and impairment, if not posttraumatic stress disorder (PTSD) or acute stress disorder (ASD). For this reason, when conditions allow—that is, if the client is not acutely psychotic, overwhelmed, or suffering from substantial cognitive impairment—the interviewer should inquire about the childhood and adulthood trauma history of those seeking psychological assistance. To some extent, how this inquiry is done is up to the interviewer, but it should minimally include general questions about major negative experiences throughout the lifespan. As described later in this chapter, such questions should be behaviorally anchored, as opposed to solely asking about "child abuse," "rape," or exposure to "disasters."

TRAUMA HISTORIES

Taking a routine trauma history may result in considerable information about important traumatic events—material that often is not volunteered without specific inquiry. For example, Briere and Zaidi (1989) surveyed the psychiatric

https://doi.org/10.1037/0000452-004
Psychological Assessment of Adult Posttraumatic States: Phenomenology, Diagnosis, and Measurement, Third Edition, by E. M. Eadie and J. Briere

emergency room (ER) medical records of 50 randomly selected women for references to a childhood history of sexual abuse and found that only 6% documented such events. In a second phase of the study, ER clinicians were requested to routinely ask patients about any history of childhood sexual victimization. When 50 medical records from this phase were examined, reference to a sexual abuse history increased more than 10-fold. Furthermore, abuse history from this second phase was associated with a wide variety of presenting problems, ranging from suicidality and substance abuse to multiple diagnoses and an increased rate of borderline personality disorder diagnoses. Although simply asking about interpersonal violence is associated with substantially higher self-reports of trauma, the clinician's overall awareness of trauma issues and knowledge of trauma-sensitive interview techniques further facilitates this process.

For example, Currier and Briere (2000) compared the amount of trauma identified by two groups of psychiatry trainees and staff: one group received a 1-hour lecture on the prevalence, impacts, and assessment of interpersonal violence, and the other received no specific information on trauma. The 167 male and female psychiatric ER patients were then evaluated by a member of one group or the other, using a standardized trauma interview. Clinicians exposed to the trauma orientation identified more sexual violence (45% vs. 24%), physical violence (74% vs. 54%), and total interpersonal violence (79% vs. 63%) than did those who did not receive the 1-hour lecture.

Single-Item Versus Multi-Item Reviews of Traumatic Events

General psychometric theory holds that a single summary item tapping a construct is often less reliable or valid than a variable composed of multiple related items (Diamantopoulos et al., 2012; Nunnally & Bernstein, 1994). For example, a single item asking whether someone is depressed may be less reliable or have less construct validity than the sum of a series of items tapping depression. This is true of trauma exposure measures as well, in which a single general item is typically less reliable in yielding accurate responses than a series of items examining specific traumatic events.

A good example of the increased reliability of multi-item measures over that of single items can be found in a study by Peirce and colleagues (2009), who compared the predictive validity of the single trauma exposure item used in the Structured Clinical Interview for *DSM-IV* (SCID; First et al., 1998) to the 17 specific trauma items of the Traumatic Life Events Questionnaire (TLEQ; Kubany et al., 2000). As Peirce et al. (2009) noted, the TLEQ "produced a 9-fold higher rate of traumatic events reported by the participants as compared to the SCID. As a result, PTSD diagnoses in the sample increased to 33% after the TLEQ measure from 24% after the SCID" (p. 210).

Described next are several multi-item trauma exposure scales that can be helpful in both (a) specifying the presence of a *Diagnostic and Statistical Manual of Mental Disorders* (*DSM*) Criterion A trauma for the diagnosis of PTSD (American Psychiatric Association, 2013, 2022) and (b) reviewing the number and type of traumatic events experienced by a client over their lifespan to date.

TRAUMA (CRITERION A) INTERVIEWS AND MEASURES

Although there are several structured clinical interviews that survey clients' trauma histories, only some of the best known are presented here. Each of these interviews evaluates a range of traumatic experiences. Some of these instruments prompt interviewer questions, whereas others are designed to be given to the client to fill out. Other *DSM* (5th ed; *DSM-5*) Criterion A instruments, not discussed here, narrowly assess in detail certain specific traumatic experiences. These include measures evaluating adult sexual assault (e.g., Koss et al., 2006), adult intimate partner violence (e.g., Shepard & Campbell, 1992; Straus, 1979), police trauma (Weiss et al., 2010), and moral injury (Norman et al., 2024). For a detailed review of Criterion A measures, the reader should consult the National Center for PTSD (2024) website.

It is important that the clinician attend to the client's reaction to the structured interview as it unfolds, so that it can be modified or even terminated if necessary. These interviews tend to move rapidly from one traumatic event to the next, typically without any formalized acknowledgment of the emotional impact of such questions or of the rapport and sensitivity required in such contexts. As a result, the interviewee may become overwhelmed or even retraumatized by the process, thereby defeating the purpose of the interview (ultimately, to help the client) as well as decreasing the quality of the interview data (e.g., by motivating avoidance or producing confusion). Although structured interviews allow for the acquisition of information in a reliable and focused manner, the clinician should see the interview items as a series of helpful prompts, rather than as a script that must be followed regardless of the respondent's distress or psychological state.

Another issue to be discussed before reviewing specific Criterion A measures is that of trauma description. Although most of the measures reviewed here provide a seemingly exhaustive list of potential stressors, not all offer behavioral descriptions of these events. Instead, they merely ask respondents to report whether, for example, they have ever been "raped," "physically assaulted," or "sexually abused as a child." Although some stressors may not require much elaboration (e.g., earthquakes or motor vehicle accidents), others—especially acts of interpersonal victimization—often must be described behaviorally before accurate assessment can occur. Hanson and colleagues (1995), for example, discussed the specific problems inherent in screening for a sexual assault history, noting the following:

> Asking respondents if they have been "raped" elicits much lower prevalence rates than if behaviorally specific structured questions are used to define sexual assault (Koss, 1983, 1993). One reason for this is that people do not always perceive a sexual assault incident to be a rape. If the assailant was a family member, a friend, or a dating partner, some individuals may not label the incident as a rape. If the assault did not involve vaginal penetration, but did involve some other type of sexual penetration (i.e., oral or anal), individuals may not categorize the event as a rape. (p. 135)

Similar to these concerns, it is not at all uncommon for a respondent to deny a history of childhood "sexual abuse" or "physical abuse" because of differing interpretations of these words. For example, some clients may not consider their sexual intercourse at age 15 with a 28-year-old boyfriend to be sexual abuse, and some respondents are known to interpret relatively extreme examples of physical maltreatment as, instead, appropriate parental discipline. Similarly, some battered women may reframe their experiences as "fighting" or "not getting along" with their partner, or they may not consider it abuse if they believe they deserved to be beaten. In some instances, this confusion appears to represent a lack of definitional understanding based on culture, geography, or gender socialization, whereas in others it is likely to arise from psychological defenses against acknowledging traumatic events.

Given this variability in response to screening items, the clinician is advised to avoid merely presenting a list of potential traumas during trauma assessment. Instead, traumatic events should be described in such a way that their definitions are unambiguous. Furthermore, brief preassessment comments regarding victimization may be helpful to the extent that they normalize or destigmatize the reporting of interpersonal violence experiences. These comments should not, however, take the form of pressuring or prescribing trauma disclosures, such that the respondent believes they *should* have something traumatic to report.

Presented next are some of the most-cited traumatic events scales and interviews. Many have been used primarily in research, although those authored by U.S. Department of Veterans Affairs (VA) staff (e.g., the Life Events Checklist for *DSM-5* [LEC-5] by Weathers et al., 2013) have been used in clinical populations as well. Even the non-VA instruments are likely to be helpful in clinical contexts.

Potential Stressful Events Interview

The Potential Stressful Events Interview (PSEI; Falsetti et al., 1994; Resnick, Falsetti, et al., 1996) is best known for its use in the fourth edition of the *DSM* (*DSM-IV*; American Psychiatric Association, 1994) PTSD field trials. Although there is no *DSM-5* (American Psychiatric Association, 2013) version of the PSEI, this interview serves as an important example of how a research measure can be useful as a clinical tool. The PSEI evaluates stressor type (divided into low and high magnitude), objective/behavioral characteristics of the stressor, and clients' subjective reactions. High-magnitude stressors evaluated include events such as war zone or combat experiences, natural disasters, childhood sexual abuse, and aggravated physical assaults. The low-magnitude stressors module evaluates events that may contribute to stress, although few would qualify as Criterion A events themselves.

There is a shorter 17-item version of the PSEI, the Trauma Assessment for Adults (TAA; Resnick, Best, et al., 1996). For each TAA item, clients are asked, among other things, their age at the time of the trauma as well as how often the trauma occurred, its duration, and whether anyone died or was hospitalized.

Stressful Life Events Screening Questionnaire

The Stressful Life Events Screening Questionnaire (SLESQ; L. A. Goodman et al., 1998) evaluates 13 traumatic events. In contrast to some measures, the SLESQ has been shown to have good test-retest reliability, adequate convergent validity, and good discrimination between Criterion A and non–Criterion A events. The authors have shown in several studies that this measure is a good predictor of posttraumatic distress and disturbance (Green et al., 2001, 2006). The SLESQ tends to focus on interpersonal traumas, about which it queries in significant detail.

Life Events Checklist for *DSM-5*

The LEC-5 by Weathers et al. (2013) was updated for the *DSM-5* from the original version by Gray et al. (2004). It examines exposure to 16 potentially traumatic events and 1 other unspecified event. The LEC-5 can be administered as a self-report or interview measure. Although it is a stand-alone measure, the LEC-5 is often administered with the Clinician-Administered PTSD Scale for *DSM-5* (CAPS-5; F. W. Weathers et al., 2018).

Traumatic Life Events Questionnaire

The TLEQ (Kubany et al., 2000) evaluates 17 potentially life-threatening events and assesses whether each traumatic event meets *DSM-IV* subjective distress Criterion A2. Although *DSM-IV* Criterion A2 is not relevant to the *DSM-5* (which dropped this criterion), this addition nevertheless provides the clinician with important information in terms of how distressing the event was perceived to be when it occurred.

Trauma History Screen

The Trauma History Screen (THS; Carlson et al., 2011) is a 14-item self-report measure that addresses similar traumas to the other measures described here. Notably, items were intentionally written at a low reading level, using common, simple language. The THS provides more information than most trauma exposure measures, including how often each event occurred, when it happened, its duration, and whether there was a threat of death or injury.

Deployment Risk and Resilience Inventory–2

The Deployment Risk and Resilience Inventory–2 (DRRI-2; Vogt et al., 2013) contains 17 separate psychometrically reliable and valid scales, tapping predeployment, deployment, and postdeployment risk and resilience factors, including a Combat Experiences Scale and a Postbattle Experiences Scale. The Combat Experiences Scale lists 17 combat experiences (e.g., "I was exposed to hostile incoming fire"), whereas the Postbattle Experiences Scale describes 13 traumatic experiences that involved witnessing war-related events (e.g., "I saw civilians after they had been severely wounded or disfigured"). Given the length of these combined scales, a brief nine-item self-report version, the Deployment Risk and Resilience Inventory–2 Warfare Exposure–Short Form (DRRI-2 WE-SF; Bovin et al., 2023), is also available. Because the DRRI-2 and its scales and short form are comprehensive and well validated, clinicians may find this suite of measures preferable to the previously published Combat Exposure Scale (Keane et al., 1989).

Broadband Trauma/Adversity Review

The Broadband Trauma/Adversity Review (BTAR; Briere, 2024) is an expansion of the Initial Trauma Review–Revised (Briere, 2004) and can be found in Appendix A (this volume). The BTAR examines 32 forms of trauma and adversity separated into those experienced before age 18 and those that occurred at age 18 or later, including child abuse and neglect, peer sexual and physical assaults, witnessing trauma, stalking, events such as motor vehicle accidents and disasters, miscarriage, torture, and police-related violence, in some cases followed by additional specific questions. The BTAR can be administered as a self-report measure or as part of a clinical interview.

Complex Trauma Questionnaire

The Complex Trauma Questionnaire (ComplexTQ; Maggiora Vergano et al., 2015) evaluates a range of early (prior to age 15 years) life adversities that have been associated with complex posttraumatic outcomes, including complex PTSD. Rated separately for maternal, paternal, and other attachment figure behaviors, the 70 items of the ComplexTQ measure lack of care (physical and emotional neglect), abuse (psychological, physical, and sexual abuse), and other experiences, such as rejection, role reversal, exposure to domestic violence, separations, and losses. There are two separate versions of the ComplexTQ, one for clinician administration and one for client self-report.

TRAUMA EXPOSURE SECTIONS WITHIN LARGER TRAUMATIC STRESS MEASURES

Two commonly used traumatic stress measures also have specific sections for assessing trauma exposure. Each is discussed next.

Harvard Trauma Questionnaire

The Harvard Trauma Questionnaire (HTQ; Mollica et al., 1992) was developed specifically for the assessment of refugees, primarily those from Indochina. However, there are now six officially translated versions of the HTQ: Vietnamese, Cambodian, Laotian, and, more recently, Japanese, Croatian, and Bosnian. The stressor section has 17 items, tapping common refugee-related traumas, including torture, rape, starvation, and exposure to the murder of others. Research on 91 refugees (Mollica et al., 1992) indicates that the stressor section is reliable, both in terms of internal consistency ($\alpha = .90$) and stability over 1 week (test-retest $r = .89$). The HTQ is a frequently cited measure of refugee traumatic experiences, both because of its structural quality and because there are few other established measures of refugee experiences (particularly torture) available.

Detailed Assessment of Posttraumatic Stress

The Detailed Assessment of Posttraumatic Stress (DAPS; Briere, 2001) includes a trauma specification module, which lists 13 potentially traumatic events. All of the DAPS events (except childhood physical abuse and childhood sexual abuse) include the requirement that the respondent was "seriously hurt or afraid [they] would be hurt or killed" (Briere, 2001).

CHILDHOOD HISTORY INTERVIEWS AND MEASURES

Most instruments that evaluate traumatic events in adulthood either overlook childhood abuse or merely include it—typically without operational definition—as one of many traumas that the respondent can endorse. There are, however, several scales that examine adult recollections of childhood maltreatment history in detail. These scales vary considerably in terms of the number of forms of abuse or neglect they assess and the amount of abuse-specific detail they offer.

Childhood Trauma Questionnaire

The Childhood Trauma Questionnaire (CTQ; D. P. Bernstein et al., 1994) is a 70-item measure that assesses childhood trauma in six areas: physical, sexual, and emotional abuse; physical and emotional neglect; and "related areas of family dysfunction (e.g., substance abuse)" (p. 1133). The CTQ is one of the most widely used abuse-exposure instruments in the child abuse literature, and this measure typically requires 10 to 15 minutes to administer. Items in the CTQ begin with the phrase "When I was growing up," and are rated on 5-point Likert-type scales. Principal component analysis of the CTQ in a sample of 286 substance-dependent patients yielded four factors that subsequently made up the scales of this measure: physical and emotional abuse, emotional neglect, sexual abuse, and physical neglect (D. P. Bernstein et al., 1997). Later analyses suggested a five-factor solution, wherein physical and emotional abuse formed separate factors (D. P. Bernstein et al., 1997; Scher et al., 2001). Because the Scher et al. (2001) study examined 1,007 community participants, the authors suggested that the means and standard deviations they reported can be considered normative data for the CTQ. There is also a 28-item short form of the CTQ, which replicates the five scales of the full measure (D. P. Bernstein et al., 2003).

Adverse Childhood Experiences Scale

The 10-item Adverse Childhood Experiences (ACEs) scale (Felitti et al., 1998) is a dichotomously scored measure of adult experiences of childhood abuse and neglect. It includes five direct exposure items (physical abuse, verbal abuse, sexual abuse, physical neglect, and emotional neglect) and five items related to adversities associated with family dysfunction (parental substance use, maternal victimization through domestic violence, a family member in jail, a family member diagnosed with a mental illness, and parental divorce, death, or abandonment). Individual items are summed to yield an overall measure of cumulative childhood adversities. The ACEs scale is widely used in public health and now in the mental health domain, and ACEs scores have been shown to be a relatively strong predictor of a range of adult outcomes, including psychological symptoms and disorders, illicit drug use and other risky behavior, suicide risk, social problems, and risk for chronic diseases.

Psychological Maltreatment Review

The Psychological Maltreatment Review (PMR; Briere et al., 2012) examines adult retrospective reports of child psychological abuse, psychological neglect, and psychological support, measured separately for maternal and paternal figures. The three scales of the PMR demonstrated good internal consistency in a sample of 1,051 members of the general population, and the structural validity of the PMR was supported by both exploratory and confirmatory factor analyses. Indicative of its construct validity, all PMR scales were significantly correlated with anxious and avoidant attachment in close relationships, partially as a function of caretaker gender. Although the PMR is—like many measures in this section—primarily used in research, its psychometric properties and large reference sample suggest its potential utility as a clinical measure of noncontact child maltreatment.

Assessing Environments III, Form SD

The Assessing Environments III, Form SD (AEIII-Form SD; Rausch & Knutson, 1991) is a revision of the AEIII, first introduced by A. M. Berger and colleagues

(1988). This scale consists of 170 items, forming the following scales: Physical Punishment, Sibling Physical Punishment, Perception of Discipline, Sibling Perception of Punishment, Deserving Punishment, and Sibling Deserving Punishment. The reliability of scales making up the SD version of the AEIII was evaluated in a sample of 421 university students, yielding KR-20 (Kuder–Richardson Formula 20) reliability coefficients ranging from .68 to .74 (Rausch & Knutson, 1991).

EXPOSURE TO SOCIAL DISCRIMINATION AND MALTREATMENT

As described in Chapter 1, maltreatment based on race, sex, ethnicity, national origin, and/or LGBTQ+ status is a significant life stressor. We describe several measures of social discrimination and maltreatment that can potentially be used to assess social adversity in clinical contexts, although only a few (e.g., the Race-Based Traumatic Stress Symptom Scale [RBTSSS]; Carter et al., 2013) have been specifically developed for clinical applications. As noted by the American Psychological Association, APA Task Force on Psychological Practice With Sexual Minority Persons (2021), clinicians "should be prepared to assess lifetime discrimination experiences, and to address an individual's reactions to these experiences in a therapeutic manner" (p. 18).

Schedule of Sexist Events

The 20-item Schedule of Sexist Events (SSE; Klonoff & Landrine, 1995) assesses various types of sexist experiences, including sexual harassment, sexist name-calling, and workplace discrimination, experienced by women over the lifespan and in the prior year. Here is an example of a typical item: "How many times have you been treated unfairly by teachers or professors because you are a woman?" The SSE is reliable and valid and SSE scores have been associated with psychological distress, behavioral health, and substance abuse (Scheer et al., 2022).

Race-Based Traumatic Stress Symptom Scale

The RBTSSS (Carter et al., 2013) is a 52-item scale that evaluates clients' emotional responses to racist experiences. Developed specifically for clinical practice, it yields seven scales (e.g., Anxiety, Depression, Hypervigilance, Avoidance, Intrusion), which are conceptualized indicators of race-based traumatic stress. The reliability and the validity of this test have been established in various studies (e.g., Pieterse et al., 2023).

Experiences of Discrimination

The Experiences of Discrimination (EOD; Krieger et al., 2005) is an 18-item measure of exposure to racial discrimination, based on an instrument used in the Coronary Artery Risk Development in Young Adults study (Krieger & Sidney, 1996). Items inquire about having ever experienced discrimination in a variety of circumstances (e.g., in school, when seeking a job, during interactions with police), how often such experiences occurred, and negative effects. The EOD is internally consistent and EOD scores are associated with psychological distress.

Daily Heterosexist Experiences Questionnaire

The Daily Heterosexist Experiences Questionnaire (DHEQ; Balsam et al., 2013) is a measure of minority stress experienced by LGBTQ+ individuals, including those who identify as nonbinary or transgender. It is composed of 50 items that form nine subscales, including Gender Expression, Vigilance, Harassment and Discrimination, and Victimization. Scores on the DHEQ have been associated with gender, sexual orientation, and psychological distress, but not race or ethnicity.

Social Discrimination and Maltreatment Scale

The 36-item Social Discrimination and Maltreatment Scale (SDMS; Briere et al., 2025) consists of three exposure subscales (Sexism, Racism, and Cis-Heterosexism) and a total score, each with severity cut-off scores. It was developed and validated in a sample of 528 adults. This measure and its subscales were internally consistent and demonstrated factorial validity in two separate subsamples. The total SDMS score was associated with *DSM-5* PTSD symptoms even when controlling for general trauma exposure, and there was a linear relationship between the number of elevated SDMS subscales and posttraumatic stress scores. A brief, 18-item version of this measure, the Social Discrimination and Maltreatment Scale—Short Form (SDMS-SF; Briere, 2023; Briere et al., 2024), with generally equivalent psychometrics, can be found in Appendix B (this volume).

CONCLUSION

What becomes clear when reviewing most trauma interviews and inventories in the field is their inherent research focus, as opposed to being specific clinical tools. Some measures provide insufficient information on a given stressor, including its behavioral definition, whereas others access far more information than would be clinically indicated. Further work in this area will be most helpful to the extent that it produces trauma review measures that are validated and reliable and that are specifically developed for clinical practice.

Most of these measures also do not include behavioral definitions for interpersonal traumas. Furthermore, because of their schematic (if not rote) interrogatory style and potential to decrease interviewer–interviewee rapport, some trauma interviews may not be immediately acceptable to the general clinical interviewer. On the other hand, these protocols tend to evaluate the full range of trauma exposure and can decrease the subjectivity and limitations of informal trauma inquiry.

5 INTERVIEWS

The majority of trauma-relevant evaluation occurs in a diagnostic interview or initial psychotherapy session, as opposed to through formal psychological testing. In fact, the occasional suggestion that emergency room or crisis center personnel consider using pencil-and-paper trauma measures is usually greeted, at best, with amusement. This reaction is contextually appropriate, in the sense that (a) trauma work often occurs in a rapid, relatively intense environment where clinical impressions are quickly formed; (b) acute trauma victims are often too distraught or distracted to attend fully to reading and writing; and (c) many mental health emergency staff are psychiatrists or social workers (i.e., they are members of disciplines that typically have less training in psychological test administration and interpretation).

Although a central tenet of this volume is that psychological testing can be very helpful in trauma assessment, it is also true that no psychological test can replace the focused attention, visible empathy, and extensive clinical experience of a well-trained and seasoned trauma clinician. As a result, it is likely that both interview-based and, when timely and appropriate, formal psychological assessments are intrinsic to a complete trauma workup. For this

https://doi.org/10.1037/0000452-005
Psychological Assessment of Adult Posttraumatic States: Phenomenology, Diagnosis, and Measurement, Third Edition, by E. M. Eadie and J. Briere

reason, this chapter focuses on issues and methodologies relevant to the diagnostic interview. Because interview-based assessments are potentially less organized and focused, however, two assessment approaches are presented here: the trauma-relevant (but informal) psychological interview and the structured diagnostic interview. As noted in Chapter 6, although these procedures can assist in the accurate specification of relevant traumatic events and formal diagnostic outcomes, such interviews cannot provide the more in-depth and normative or comparative information generated from comprehensive psychological testing. Thus, it is recommended that structured, interview-based assessment be seen as an important tool but not as a procedure that necessarily obviates the (often later) need for psychological test data.

Finally, the description of structured interviews in this chapter is not meant to suggest that such instruments are necessary in all instances or for all interviewers. Some clinical settings and situations do not require the detailed assessment provided by structured interviews, and some trauma-specialized clinicians feel themselves to be sufficiently conversant with the relevant criteria and issues that they do not require the prompts of a structured procedure. On the other hand, research suggests that routine clinical diagnosis (i.e., without a formal structured interview) may miss as many as half of all actual cases of posttraumatic stress disorder (PTSD; Zimmerman & Mattia, 1999). Even highly experienced trauma clinicians can benefit from the use of structured interviews on occasion, such as in certain forensic or research contexts, or when diagnostic issues are especially complex, as in the assessment and diagnosis of dissociative disorders (Bailey et al., 2019).

THE TRAUMA-RELEVANT ASSESSMENT INTERVIEW

In most mental health clinics and psychiatric emergency rooms, the assessment of psychological disturbance occurs during the diagnostic interview or mental status examination. In the interview session, the client is typically evaluated for the following:

- altered consciousness or mental functioning (i.e., for evidence of dementia, confusion, delirium, cognitive impairment, or other organic disturbance),
- psychotic symptoms (e.g., hallucinations, delusions, thought disorder, disorganized behavior, or "negative" signs),
- evidence of self-injurious or suicidal thoughts and behaviors,
- potential danger to others,
- mood disturbance (i.e., depression, anxiety),

- substance abuse or addiction, and
- personality dysfunction.

In combination with other information (e.g., from the client, significant others, and outside agencies), these interview data provide the basis for diagnosis and an intervention plan.

Because these clinical issues are frequently of immediate importance, assessment for other disorders or dysfunctional states often is postponed or deferred entirely. However, if the presenting problem is a posttraumatic reaction, these standard clinical screens miss important information. The following list describes the key elements to be investigated in a clinical interview when there is the possibility of trauma-related disturbance. Although some settings will require a brief inquiry, the interviewer should explore the following symptom areas in sufficient detail (when time allows and the client is sufficiently stable) to determine their absence or presence, frequency or severity, and impact on functioning.

- Symptoms of Posttraumatic Stress
  - Intrusive experiences such as flashbacks, nightmares, reliving experiences, or intrusive thoughts and memories
  - Avoidant symptoms such as behavioral or cognitive attempts to avoid trauma-reminiscent stimuli, as well as emotional numbing
  - Hyperarousal symptoms such as decreased or restless sleep, muscle tension, irritability, jumpiness, or attention and concentration difficulties
  - Alteration in mood (e.g., depression) or cognitions (e.g., self-blame) related to the trauma(s)

- Dissociative Responses
  - Depersonalization or derealization experiences
  - Fugue states
  - "Spacing out" or cognitive-emotional disengagement
  - Amnesia or missing time
  - Identity alteration or confusion

- Somatic Disturbance
  - Conversion reactions (e.g., paralysis, anesthesia, blindness, deafness)
  - Somatization (i.e., excessive preoccupation with bodily dysfunction)
  - Psychogenic pain (e.g., pelvic pain, chronic pain)

- Sexual Disturbance (especially secondary to sexual abuse or adult assault)
  - Sexual distress, including sexual dysfunction
  - Sexual fears and conflicts
- Trauma-Related Cognitive Disturbance
  - Low self-esteem and self-critical beliefs
  - Helplessness
  - Hopelessness
  - Overvalued ideas regarding the level of threat or danger in the environment
  - Irrational guilt and self-blame
- Distress-Reduction Behaviors
  - Self-injury
  - Bingeing and/or purging
  - Excessive or impulsive sexual behavior
  - Compulsive stealing
  - Impulsive or reactive aggression
  - Excessive risk-taking
- Transient Posttraumatic Psychotic Reactions
  - Trauma-related loosened associations
  - Trauma-related hallucinations (often trauma congruent)
  - Trauma-related delusions (often trauma congruent, especially paranoia)
- Culture-Specific Trauma Responses (when appropriate). Some examples are as follows:
  - *Ataque de nervios* ("attack of nerves" in Latin American culture)
  - *Khyâl* (panic-like attacks in Cambodian culture)
  - *Susto* (an illness attributed to a frightening event in some Latin American cultures)

This list is more comprehensive than is indicated for certain posttraumatic presentations (e.g., a survivor of a motor vehicle accident), although most or all of the components may be relevant for certain chronic traumas (e.g., extended child abuse or torture). Some version of this examination is usually indicated, however, even if it is followed by a more structured diagnostic interview, because it evaluates specific symptoms, behaviors, and clinical issues, as opposed to solely the presence or absence of psychological disorders.

STRUCTURED DIAGNOSTIC INTERVIEWS

Structured diagnostic interviews are used primarily to generate objectively determined *Diagnostic and Statistical Manual of Mental Disorders (DSM)* diagnoses. By providing the examiner with a list of diagnostic criteria and specific questions to tap those criteria, such interviews ideally decrease the chance of diagnostic error and increase the likelihood of covering all relevant symptoms. This may especially be the case when the client presents with a complex trauma history and a range of significant posttraumatic stress, behavioral, and dissociative symptoms. For this reason, we strongly suggest the use of validated structured diagnostic interviews over more informal clinical interviews.

Posttraumatic Stress Disorder Interviews

As noted in Chapter 2 (this volume), the diagnostic criteria of the fifth edition of the *DSM* and its text revision (*DSM-5* & *DSM-5-TR*; American Psychiatric Association, 2013, 2022) for PTSD and acute stress disorder (ASD) no longer require that all symptoms be specifically associated with one index trauma. This is a welcome update, because it more closely aligns with many trauma survivors' actual experiences of multiple adversities and more complex symptom presentation (Karam et al., 2014). Nevertheless, most of the interviews reviewed next continue to require that posttraumatic symptoms be directly linked to one specific trauma.

There are several structured interviews that allow the clinician to render a diagnosis of PTSD with reasonable confidence. Presented next are the best known and most validated of these.

Clinician-Administered Posttraumatic Stress Disorder Scale for *DSM-5*

The Clinician-Administered Posttraumatic Stress Disorder Scale for *DSM-5* (CAPS-5; F. W. Weathers, Blake, et al., 2013) is considered by many to be the gold standard structured interview for PTSD. It is an updated version of the CAPS (Blake et al., 1990, 1995), originally developed to assess PTSD as set out in the revised third edition of the *DSM* (*DSM-III-R*) and then in the fourth edition (*DSM-IV*) and revised to correspond to *DSM-5* criteria (American Psychiatric Association, 1987, 1994, 2013).

The interview is composed of 30 items, assessing for the 20 PTSD symptoms in the *DSM-5* as well as the onset and duration of symptoms, subjective distress, impact on social and occupational functioning, overall response validity, overall symptom severity, and items addressing the dissociative sub-type of PTSD (i.e., derealization and depersonalization). The CAPS-5 has several useful features, including standard prompts, follow-up questions, and explicit, behaviorally anchored rating scales. Item severity is rated on a 5-point Likert scale (0 = *absent* to 4 = *extreme/incapacitating*), which is a simplification from the prior version that assessed item frequency and intensity separately. The interview can be used to assess for a current (*past month*) or lifetime (*worst month*) diagnosis of PTSD and to measure PTSD symptoms over the past week. For diagnostic purposes, a DSM-5 symptom criterion is considered met if an item is rated as 2 (*moderate/threshold*) or greater in severity.

The CAPS-5 is one of the structured interviews that requires identification of a single Criterion A index trauma. This index trauma can consist of a single incident or multiple, closely related incidents (e.g., "the worst parts of your combat experiences"). For symptoms that are not obviously tied to the index trauma (e.g., "reckless or self-destructive behavior"), the interviewer must indicate the level of *trauma-relatedness* attributing that symptom to the index event. Whereas the CAPS for *DSM-IV* allowed for endorsement of up to three traumatic events that were then considered in the evaluation of symptoms, the CAPS-5 typically relies on just one index trauma. This simplifies administration but potentially at the cost of assessing for symptom experiences that relate to traumas other than the index event. It is recommended that the Life Events Checklist for *DSM-5* (LEC-5; Weathers et al., 2013) be administered alongside the CAPS-5.

Psychometric data for the CAPS-5 are encouraging (F. W. Weathers et al., 2018). In a validation study with 374 military veterans, the CAPS-5 had good test-retest reliability and interrater reliability for both diagnostic status ($r = .83$; $K = .78$, respectively) and total severity ($r = .78$; intraclass correlation coefficient [ICC] = .91, respectively). The total score also showed high internal consistency ($\alpha = .88$), and the measure overall demonstrated good convergent and discriminant validity. Of note, the CAPS-5 corresponds closely to the prior version of the interview (CAPS for *DSM-IV*), allowing continuity when assessing for PTSD across *DSM* editions.

Structured Clinical Interview for *DSM-5*

The Structured Clinical Interview for *DSM-5* (SCID-5; First et al., 2016) is one of the most widely used diagnostic interview systems. The SCID-5 consists of several modules corresponding to the major diagnostic categories in the *DSM-5*. Module L is used to assess for PTSD, ASD, adjustment disorder, and other specified trauma- and stressor-related disorders. Updates from the prior version of the SCID include a simplified series of questions to assess for exposure to a broader range of traumatic events and removal of the screening question that allowed the module to be skipped if it was not endorsed. Responses are coded as *absent, present,* or *subthreshold.* As a result, a continuous symptom severity score is not available with this measure. PTSD status can be determined for the present (past month) or for the individual's lifetime and is made based on the PTSD diagnostic algorithm.

The SCID-5 has the advantage of screening for a variety of disorders in addition to PTSD. However, the SCID-5 does not assess for dissociative disorders; this can be problematic when the client is experiencing significant dissociative symptomatology, because the interview inquires about symptoms often attributed to dissociation, such as hearing voices related to dissociative identity disorder (DID), or emotional or physical nonresponsiveness. In such cases, the absence of a dissociative disorders option can lead to these symptoms being incorrectly attributed to a psychotic disorder (Brand, 2024). Beyond this concern, however, the SCID-5's broad diagnostic range provides a more comprehensive clinical picture than is available with most trauma-specific measures, and it supports assessment of relevant comorbidities. Although the SCID-5 appears to be a rigorous interview assessment tool that has good preliminary psychometric characteristics (e.g., Shabani et al., 2021), further validation of this interview (especially Module L) is indicated.

Structured Interview for Posttraumatic Stress Disorder
The Structured Interview for Posttraumatic Stress Disorder (SI-PTSD; J. Davidson et al., 1989) consists of 17 items designed to tap *DSM-IV* PTSD criteria as well as two items to assess guilt. It has not yet been updated for the *DSM-5*. Items are rated on a 5-point severity scale (0 = *absent* to 4 = *extremely severe*) and are endorsed for both current and lifetime (*worst ever*) status. Symptoms must be rated as a 2 (*moderate*) or higher to meet PTSD criteria.

In a sample of veterans (Davidson et al., 1989), the SI-PTSD had very good internal consistency (α = .94) and good sensitivity and specificity with regard to the SCID-PTSD (.96 and .80, respectively, yielding a K of .79). In a clinical sample (Davidson, Book, et al., 1997), the SI-PTSD showed strong interrater reliability and good test-retest reliability.

Posttraumatic Stress Disorder Symptom Scale–Interviewer for *DSM-5*
The Posttraumatic Stress Disorder Symptom Scale–Interviewer for *DSM-5* (PSSI-5; Foa et al., 2016b) is a 24-item semistructured interview that assesses *DSM-5* symptoms of PTSD as well as level of distress and interference with functioning over the past month. The interview begins with an inquiry about

exposure to Criterion A events and, in the case of multiple identified events, the index trauma is identified by selecting the "traumatic event that is currently most distressing" (Foa et al., 2016b).

Items are rated on a scale of frequency and severity ranging from 0 (*not at all*) to 4 (*6 or more times per week/severe*). A symptom is considered to be present for diagnostic purposes if it is rated a 1 (*once a week or less/a little*) or higher. A sum of the 20 PTSD symptoms also yields an overall severity score. The instrument was validated with a sample of 242 trauma-exposed college undergraduates, veterans, and residents of an urban community recruited from three separate sites (Foa et al., 2016a,b). The PSSI-5 showed good convergent and discriminant validity, strong test-retest reliability ($r = .87$), and interrater agreement, as well as good internal consistency ($\alpha = .89$) for the symptom severity score. The authors recommend a cutoff score of 23 to determine a probable PTSD diagnosis.

Anxiety and Related Disorders Interview Schedule for *DSM-5*

An updated version of the Anxiety and Related Disorders Interview Schedule (ADIS-5; T. A. Brown & Barlow, 2014) was developed to correspond with *DSM-5*. This structured interview assesses for mood and anxiety disorders and several related disorders, including PTSD and ASD, with versions for current symptoms and lifetime occurrence. Other presenting concerns such as eating disorders, dissociation, and psychosis are screened for but not fully assessed. The section on PTSD includes a systematic inquiry of trauma exposure, adding more structure over the previously open-ended question on the ADIS-IV (T. A. Brown et al., 1994) and earlier versions. There has been little research on the psychometric qualities of the ADIS-5. The prior version was used in several clinical research studies (Barlow et al., 2017; T. A. Brown et al., 2001; Erwin et al., 2002).

Other Structured Interviews

In addition to those for PTSD, structured clinical interviews are available to assess other posttraumatic outcomes. These include interviews for ASD, the dissociative disorders, and complex PTSD.

Structured Interview for Disorders of Extreme Stress—Revised

The Structured Interview for Disorders of Extreme Stress—Revised (SIDES-R; Pelcovitz et al., 1997) was originally developed as a companion to existing interview-based rating scales for PTSD. The first edition of the SIDES measured current and lifetime indicators of disorders of extreme stress, not otherwise specified (DESNOS; van der Kolk et al., 2005), an early version of what is now considered complex PTSD. The SIDES was first revised by Ford and Kidd (1998), with some item rewordings but no changes to the overall scoring procedures. A more substantial revision was conducted by Scoboria and colleagues (2008), who shortened the interview and derived a new factor structure.

The SIDES-R contains five factor scales: Demoralization, Somatic Dysregulation, Anger Dysregulation, Risk/Self-Harm, and Altered Sexuality. Scores on the SIDES-R are associated with early traumatic experiences, interpersonal trauma, and prolonged traumatic exposure. However, this interview does not directly assess for trauma exposure and symptoms are not necessarily linked to a specific traumatic experience. Although the SIDES is typically employed as a measure of complex PTSD, it should be noted that the SIDES does not systematically evaluate the symptom criteria for PTSD as set out in the *DSM-5*. Both the original SIDES and the newer SIDES-R demonstrate acceptable internal consistency and good construct validity (Pelcovitz et al., 1997; Scoboria et al., 2008).

Acute Stress Disorder Structured Interview–5

The Acute Stress Disorder Structured Interview–5 (ASDI-5; Bryant, 2016) is the updated version of the ASDI (Bryant et al., 1998) and is a useful tool when the diagnostic question pertains to ASD rather than PTSD. This interview evaluates each of the intrusive, mood-related, dissociative, effortful avoidance, and arousal symptoms of ASD, along with the other criteria laid out in the *DSM-5*. The ASDI-5 is straightforward and can be administered in a relatively short period of time. Because symptoms are dichotomously scored (yes or no), severity of ASD cannot be determined. The ASDI-5 does not include a systematic assessment of trauma event exposures and, instead, can be accompanied by one of the measures in Chapter 4 for that purpose.

The original ASDI showed good reliability and validity, and it had high sensitivity and specificity (.91 and .93, respectively) with reference to clinicians' ASD diagnoses using *DSM-IV* criteria (Bryant et al., 1998). The updated ASDI-5 has not yet been validated.

Dissociative Disorders Interview Schedule

The Dissociative Disorders Interview Schedule (DDIS; Ross, 1997; Ross et al., 1989) is a structured interview with 131 items that assess for the dissociative disorders, along with borderline personality disorder, somatic symptom disorder, depression, psychotic symptoms, extrasensory experiences, and substance abuse. Respondents are also asked about a history of childhood physical or sexual abuse. Items and scoring instructions have been updated to be consistent with *DSM-5* diagnostic criteria (Ross, n.d.). The DDIS appears to be sensitive to the diagnosis of DID but there are little validity or diagnostic utility data available for other dissociative diagnoses. In a study of psychiatric inpatients, Ross and colleagues (2002) found good chance-corrected agreement (K = .74) between the DDIS and the SCID-D (described next) in identifying DID or Dissociative Disorder Not Otherwise Specified (DDNOS). There is also a self-report version of the DDIS available with good agreement to the interview version (Ross & Browning, 2016).

Semi-Structured Clinical Interview for Dissociative Symptoms and Disorders

The Semi-Structured Clinical Interview for Dissociative Symptoms and Disorders (SCID-D; Steinberg, 1994, 2023) is an interactive, semistructured interview that evaluates dissociative symptoms and disorders according to a five-component model of dissociation composed of amnesia, depersonalization, derealization, identity confusion, and identity alteration. Also evaluated by the SCID-D are observable "intra-interview dissociative cues," such as alterations in demeanor, spontaneous age regression, and trancelike appearance, which are coded in a postinterview section. The interview follows a similar format as the SCID-5 and can be used as an additional module or a standalone instrument. The reliability, validity, and diagnostic utility of the SCID-D have been demonstrated in several studies (for a meta-analytic review, see Mychailyszyn et al., 2021).

The newest version of the SCID-D (Steinberg, 2023) retains the same interview questions, reportedly preserves the psychometric properties of previous versions, and generates a symptom profile and separate scoresheets that are available for both the *DSM-5-TR* and the *International Statistical Classification of Diseases and Related Health Problems, Eleventh Revision* (*ICD-11*; World Health Organization, 2022). Subject to additional positive evaluation, the newest *DSM-5* version of the SCID-D will likely replace the prior (*DSM-IV*) SCID-D as the gold standard for interview-based assessment of dissociative disorders.

Clinician-Administered Dissociative States Scale

The Clinician-Administered Dissociative States Scale (CADSS; Bremner et al., 1998) is a unique measure among dissociation tests, because it evaluates present-state dissociation and it includes both client and clinician or observer components. For example, consider this typical client report item: "(At this time, in this room) . . . (d)o things seem to be moving in slow motion?" Here is a representative observer item: "Did the subject blank out or space out, or in some other way appear to have lost track of what was going on?"

Psychometric analysis of the CADSS in a mixed group of participants indicated strong interrater agreement (ICC = .92) and internal consistency (α = .90) on the observer items as well as high internal consistency (α = .94) on the client report items. Moderate correlations were found between the CADSS and the DES (r = .48) and SCID-D (r = .42). A more recent validation study with the German version of the CADSS (Mertens & Daniels, 2022) found similar levels of reliability and convergent validity as well as a three-factor solution consisting of depersonalization/derealization, identity confusion/alteration, and amnesia factors. Although the clinical utility of measuring state dissociation may be less obvious than measurement of trait-level dissociation, the CADSS authors noted this may be a particularly useful way to assess an individual's response to treatment (Bremner et al., 1998).

Depersonalization Severity Scale
The six-item Depersonalization Severity Scale (DSS; Simeon et al., 2001) is a brief clinician-administered scale in which the evaluator assigns a severity value for each item (0 = *none* to 3 = *severe*) based on the client's response. In a sample of 63 individuals, the DSS had low to moderate internal consistency (α = .59), but excellent interrater reliability (r = .98 for the total score), good convergent validity, and evidence of sensitivity as a measure of treatment effects. Although the DSS appears to be a useful and efficient tool for assessing depersonalization symptoms, further research on its psychometric qualities is indicated.

CONCLUSION

A number of interviews are available to assist the clinician in the standardized assessment and diagnosis of PTSD, ASD, and dissociative disorders. Several of these have only recently been updated to *DSM-5* criteria and do not yet have substantial data regarding their diagnostic utility for current *DSM* diagnoses.

Generally, it appears that the CAPS-5 and SCID-5 interviews are most helpful in diagnosing PTSD, with some slight trade-off between the two measures. The CAPS-5 is probably the most accurate of the two vis-à-vis a *DSM-5* diagnosis of PTSD, whereas the SCID-5 is able to provide diagnostic information on other potentially comorbid disorders, with the exception of dissociative disorders. To assess for dissociative diagnoses, the Semi-Structured Clinical Interview for Dissociative Symptoms and Disorders (SCID-D) should be administered alongside the SCID-5. If time is limited, the PSSI-5 has a shorter administration time than the CAPS-5, with comparable psychometric properties (Foa & Tolin, 2000). Those needing to assess for ASD have the option of using either the SCID-5 or the ASDI-5. Of the two, the ASDI-5 is more comprehensive, although the SCID-5 has the advantage of assessing ASD alongside a range of disorders. Finally, the SIDES-R is currently the only valid structured interview to assess more complex posttraumatic outcomes (i.e., complex PTSD).

Deciding which interview to administer is a multifaceted task and may involve consideration of the extent to which the client can tolerate detailed and systematic face-to-face assessment, the amount of time available, the specific goals of assessment, and, in some cases, the interviewer's level of skill and experience. When an accurate and defensible *DSM-5-TR* diagnosis is most important (e.g., in some research and forensic contexts), highly structured and comprehensive interviews are usually best. When the assessment occurs in more general clinical contexts, however, the evaluator is advised to use whatever method best fits the demands of the clinical situation. In some cases, this too will mean use of instruments such as the CAPS-5 or SCID-5; in others (e.g., when the client is especially stressed, easily overwhelmed, or time is limited), only a cursory diagnostic evaluation may be possible. When the level of evaluation is significantly reduced, however, the clinician should indicate in the assessment report any possible effect on (including decreased confidence in) the final assessment product.

6 GENERIC MEASURES

In contrast to interview-based measures, objective and projective/performance-based measures rely on individuals' responses to stimuli that do not arise from the clinical interview process. In this chapter, several major objective tests and one performance-based instrument (the Rorschach) are described in terms of their sensitivity to, and assessment of, posttraumatic states. In some instances, these tests contain no trauma-specific items or scales. In others, special items or scoring approaches have been included. Standardized psychological tests have the advantage of providing normative comparisons, often have objective indicators of response style, and can cover a breadth of content beyond what is typically assessed in a clinical interview. Combining a trauma-focused interview with test data generally results in a more comprehensive and robust trauma assessment.

MINNESOTA MULTIPHASIC PERSONALITY INVENTORY

The Minnesota Multiphasic Personality Inventory (MMPI; Hathaway & McKinley, 1943), the MMPI-2 (Butcher et al., 1989), and the MMPI-2–Restructured Form (MMPI-2-RF; Ben-Porath & Tellegen, 2008) have been

https://doi.org/10.1037/0000452-006
Psychological Assessment of Adult Posttraumatic States: Phenomenology, Diagnosis, and Measurement, Third Edition, by E. M. Eadie and J. Briere

used in a number of studies to assess posttraumatic states and disturbance. Research using the most recent version, the MMPI-3 (Ben-Porath & Tellegen, 2020), is still in the early stages of dissemination at the time of this writing, although it will eventually contribute to our understanding of how the MMPI can be used in the assessment of posttraumatic states. As a result, this section primarily considers research findings and guidance from the MMPI-2 and the MMPI-2-RF, with reference to the MMPI-3 where relevant.

Minnesota Multiphasic Personality Inventory Validity Scales

As discussed in Chapter 3, one of the primary uses of MMPI validity scales in trauma and posttraumatic stress disorder (PTSD) assessment is to measure an individual's response style and the validity of the assessment results. Unfortunately, however, trauma survivors tend to have elevated scores on standard MMPI and MMPI-2-RF validity scales relative to other clinical groups (Franklin, Repasky, et al., 2002; Frueh et al., 2000; Goodwin et al., 2013). As a result, some trauma survivors and PTSD sufferers may be seen as intentionally overreporting their symptoms when, in fact, they are accurately reporting trauma-relevant experiences, comorbidities, and unusually high psychological distress (Engelhard et al., 2007; Franklin, Rapasky, et al., 2002). In a similar vein, those with trauma-related dissociation are more likely to endorse items on validity scales that overlap with true dissociative symptoms (e.g., Brand et al., 2016).

Fortunately, it appears that several MMPI-2 validity indicators, although elevated for trauma survivors, are even more elevated for those who intentionally overreport (Arbisi, 2006; Garcia et al., 2010; Wetter et al., 1993). This is especially true for the F scales (F-K index and Fp, in particular) as well as the Dissimulation (Ds) scale. The Fp scale was developed to address the fact that individuals with high levels of psychopathology tend to score highly on the F scale and thus may be inappropriately seen as malingering. Because those with PTSD often endorse a fair amount of general (i.e., not PTSD-specific) symptomatology on the MMPI, it would be reasonable to assume that the Fp scale might be better than the F scale in detecting valid versus invalid PTSD profiles. This assumption was born out in two studies, wherein the Fp scale demonstrated greater sensitivity than the F scale in discriminating valid from invalid PTSD protocols (Elhai, Gold, Sellers, et al., 2001; Elhai et al., 2002).

Based on the partial success of the Fp scale in controlling for psychopathology while still detecting valid versus invalid MMPI responses, the Infrequency-Posttraumatic Stress Disorder scale (Fptsd; Elhai et al., 2002) was developed. The Fptsd scale attempts to measure overreporting while simultaneously avoiding the usual elevation of validity scales in the presence of posttraumatic stress. Created from MMPI-2 items that were rarely endorsed by male combat veterans in a large U.S. Department of Veterans Affairs (VA) sample, this scale was significantly less related to psychopathology and distress and was better at discriminating simulated from actual PTSD than other MMPI validity scales. The MMPI-2 Fptsd scale has not yet been updated for the MMPI-2-RF or MMPI-3. When trauma-related dissociation is the primary presentation, a number of studies have demonstrated that MMPI-2 validity indices can differentiate between individuals with genuine dissociative identity disorder and those who are feigning (Ambrose et al., 2025; Brand et al., 2016).

Minnesota Multiphasic Personality Inventory Posttraumatic Stress Disorder Scales and Profiles

One of the considerations in using broadband self-report inventories to assess posttraumatic psychopathology is that PTSD and other trauma-related presentations are quite heterogeneous, with symptoms spanning several domains of psychopathology. Because the *Diagnostic and Statistical Manual of Mental Disorders, Fifth Edition, Text Revision* (*DSM-5-TR*) criteria (American Psychiatric Association, 2022) for PTSD are divided into four separate symptom clusters (reexperiencing, avoidance, negative cognitions and mood, and hyperarousal; Chapter 2, this volume), it is not uncommon for symptoms from each cluster to be represented by different clinical scales on a measure like the MMPI (Kremyar et al., 2023).

Using the code-type approach from the MMPI-2, one of the most common 2-point profiles of PTSD sufferers is an 8-2. This profile involves elevations on the Schizophrenia (Sc) and Depression (D) scales, along with a high F scale (Fairbank et al., 1983; Keane et al., 1984; Munley et al., 1995; J. P. Wilson & Walker, 1990). PTSD sufferers also sometimes endorse scale 7 (Psychasthenia [Pt]; Lucenko et al., 2000; Rademaker et al., 2009). Other clinical scales are often elevated above T65 or T70 as well, typically generating a variety of 3-point profiles but no definitive code type (Forbes et al., 1999; Munley et al., 1995; Rademaker et al., 2009; Scheibe et al., 2001).

The MMPI-2-RF and the MMPI-3 are structured differently from the MMPI-2, resulting in different profiles for trauma-exposed individuals. These more recent versions rely on hierarchically arranged sets of scales, including the Higher-Order (H-O), Restructured Clinical (RC), and Specific Problem (SP) scales. On the H-O scales, PTSD is consistently associated with an elevation on the Emotional/Internalizing Dysfunction scale (Ben-Porath & Tellegen, 2020; Kremyar et al., 2023). On the RC scales, elevations differ somewhat by PTSD symptom cluster, with RC7 (Dysfunctional Negative Emotions) predicting reexperiencing, avoidance, and hyperarousal symptoms. The Somatic Complaints (RC1) and Aberrant Experiences (RC8) scales tend to be associated with reexperiencing symptoms, whereas Demoralization (RCd) shows the strongest prediction of PTSD Criterion D symptoms, especially mood-related cognitions (Kremyar et al., 2023). Overall, although the various MMPI tests are useful tools to assess the broad range and severity of symptoms associated with trauma, a definitive posttraumatic code type or profile has not emerged (Rademaker et al., 2009).

For the most part, the validity scales on the MMPI-2-RF are similarly effective in detecting symptom exaggeration or feigning relative to those on the MMPI-2, with the MMPI-2-RF scales having no significant advantage over the MMPI-2 (Aparcero et al., 2023). In general, of the three most recent versions of the MMPI, the MMPI-2-RF Validity (and Clinical) scales may be the least preferred choices relative to the MMPI-3 and the MMPI-2.

Minnesota Multiphasic Personality Inventory–3 Scales
The newest version, MMPI-3, does not include a PTSD scale. Instead, the Anxiety-Related Experiences (ARX) scale from the Specific Problems scales offers the closest approximation of PTSD symptomatology. There is some early empirical support that the ARX scale is predictive of PTSD symptom clusters on the Detailed Assessment of Posttraumatic Stress (DAPS; Kremyar et al., 2023) and on other self-report measures of trauma-related symptoms (Keen et al., 2024), albeit with more modest correlations in the latter instance. It includes 15 items and appears to have incremental predictive utility over the Anxiety (AXY) scale from the MMPI-2-RF (Keen et al., 2024). At the same time, however, the ARX offers fewer options for the assessment of posttraumatic symptoms on the MMPI-3 compared with its predecessor, the MMPI-2, which has two scoreable PTSD scales.

Minnesota Multiphasic Personality Inventory–2 Scales
The MMPI-2 assesses PTSD symptoms through the PS (Schlenger & Kulka, 1989) and PK (Keane et al., 1984) scales. Although the PS has good internal consistency and discriminates between research participants with and without PTSD, the PK is used more often and may be somewhat more predictive of PTSD (Munley et al., 1995). The PK scale, developed by Keane and colleagues (1984) for the MMPI, was revised slightly for the MMPI-2. The original MMPI version was validated on a sample of 200 male combat veterans (100 with PTSD and 100 diagnosed with psychiatric disorders other than PTSD), wherein 49 items were found to maximally discriminate PTSD

status. Based on visual inspection of the distribution of scores on the PK, it was determined that a raw score of 30 was the best cutoff for discriminating PTSD from other psychiatric diagnoses. This cutoff score yielded a hit rate (i.e., correct prediction percentage) of 82% in the original validation sample. Other studies have since verified the predictive validity of the original PK scale (e.g., Koretzky & Peck, 1990; Litz et al., 1991; Orr et al., 1990; Watson et al., 1994), although cutoffs as low as 19 to 23 have been recommended (e.g., D. Herman et al., 1993; Koretzky & Peck, 1990). Although the PK scale appears to be valid even when administered as a stand-alone measure (D. Herman et al., 1993; Scotti et al., 1996), it is probably most helpful in the context of other MMPI scores.

The MMPI-2 version of the PK scale has 46 items rather than the 49 contained in the MMPI version. This version was standardized on the MMPI-2 normative sample and thus generates *T*-scores based on 2,600 research participants from the general population (Lyons & Keane, 1992). In the normative sample analysis, the PK had α reliabilities of .86 and .89 for males and females, respectively, with a suggested cutoff of 28. Using this new cutoff score, Munley et al. (1995) found the PK to have a 76% hit rate for PTSD in a sample of 54 VA patients. Several other studies also indicate that the MMPI-2 PK scale discriminates those with PTSD from those without (e.g., Forbes et al., 1999; Koretzky & Peck, 1990; Perrin et al., 1997). There has been some criticism of the PK scale, however. Among the concerns are (a) it was developed and validated in primarily veteran samples and thus it may be more sensitive to war-related PTSD than to PTSD arising from civilian traumas; (b) there is a possibility that the 30- or 28-point PK scale cutoffs (MMPI and MMPI-2, respectively) are too high (for review, see Norris & Hamblen, 2004); (c) there is a likelihood that the PK discriminates trauma exposure as much as (or more than) PTSD per se; and (d) there is a wide variety of non–PTSD-like symptom items (as opposed to the small number of PTSD-specific items) contained in the scales, which can potentially produce false-positive results when applied to depressed or highly symptomatic (but not traumatized) individuals (e.g., Wetzel et al. 2003).

Minnesota Multiphasic Personality Inventory Dissociation Scales

Less developed than the MMPI scales measuring posttraumatic stress are those attempting to tap dissociation. There is no defining code type and no scales are specifically designed to measure dissociation symptoms in any MMPI version. However, individuals with severe dissociation tend to score highly on scale 8 (Schizophrenia [Sc]) with additional elevations often found on scales 6 (Paranoia), 2 (Depression), 7 (Psychasthenia), and 4 (Psychopathic Deviate; Brand, 2024; Brand & Chasson, 2015; Elhai, Gold, Mateus, et al., 2001). On scale 8, in particular, many of the items directly tap dissociative symptoms and trauma-related experiences (Brand et al., 2016).

Although several MMPI or MMPI-2 dissociation scales have been devised (e.g., Leavitt, 2001; Mann, 1995; D. W. Phillips, 1994; Sanders, 1986), few have sufficient psychometric data (especially evidence of cross-validation in other samples) to justify their general clinical use at this time. Part of the problem is that dissociation was not a focus of MMPI item writers; thus, the construct is not sufficiently addressed within the item set, making it difficult to generate a robust dissociation scale, including on the MMPI-3.

MILLON CLINICAL MULTIAXIAL INVENTORY

The Millon Clinical Multiaxial Inventory (MCMI; Millon, 1983), MCMI-II (Millon, 1987), MCMI-III (Millon, 1994), and MCMI-IV (Millon et al., 2015) are among the most popular of personality tests. However, the MCMIs are primarily used to assess personality functioning, with clinical syndromes as a secondary focus. Despite being published in 2015, the peer-reviewed literature on the newest version (the MCMI-IV) is still quite limited, requiring clinicians to rely on research from the prior versions of the test. Although the MCMI-IV includes a PTSD scale, it may have limited utility if the primary goal of an assessment is to specifically measure symptoms of posttraumatic stress.

Millon Clinical Multiaxial Inventory Profiles Related to Trauma Exposure Type

Studies employing the MCMI scales with adult trauma survivors have been conducted mostly with combat veterans, with fewer studies of other trauma populations. Earlier research suggests that those suffering posttraumatic stress may have elevations on some combination of the Avoidant, Schizoid, Passive-Aggressive, and Borderline Personality Disorder scales, along with (in many cases) the Anxiety and Dysthymia Clinical Syndrome scales (e.g., Hyer et al., 1990; Munley et al., 1995). Studies using earlier versions of the MCMI with physical and sexual abuse survivors (e.g., J. G. Allen et al., 1998; Busby et al., 1993; Fisher et al., 1993) reported scores in the clinical range on a variety of MCMI scales, and these individuals were most likely to have elevations on the Avoidant, Dependent, Passive-Aggressive, and Borderline Personality scales, along with the following Clinical Scales: Anxiety, Somatoform, Thought Disorder, Major Depression, and Delusional Disorder.

A potential problem associated with interpreting trauma survivor responses to the MCMI is whether high scores on a given scale indicate that the survivor, in fact, "has" the relevant disorder or personality style. For example, clinical experience suggests that most abuse survivors who have elevated scores on the MCMI Thought Disorder or Delusional Disorder scales do not have clinically significant psychotic symptoms, nor do all of those with an elevated Borderline scale score necessarily have borderline personality disorder. In the latter instance, the MCMI Borderline scale may be elevated by the distress reduction behaviors and interpersonal difficulties associated with childhood maltreatment. Similarly, the MCMI Psychotic scales (like the Rorschach in various trauma contexts) can tap posttraumatic symptoms, especially intrusion, avoidance, and dissociation, as well as the chaotic internal experience associated with severe abuse. Jon G. Allen and colleagues (1997) found a strong association between the Dissociative Experiences Scale (DES; E. M. Bernstein & Putnam, 1986) and the Thought Disorder scale on the MCMI-III in a group of trauma-exposed female inpatients. The authors suggested that severely dissociative trauma survivors may lose the ability to differentiate between internal experiences and external intrusions, leading to more reporting of hallucinations and delusions as well as difficulty with reality testing.

Assessing Posttraumatic Stress Disorder on the Millon Clinical Multiaxial Inventory

One reason the MCMI was underapplied to trauma survivors was the absence of a PTSD scale in that version and in the MCMI-II. Lacking such a scale, PTSD symptoms were easily misinterpreted as evidence of personality dysfunction (e.g., borderline personality or, before the MCMI-III, the construct of "self-defeating" personality). Choca et al. (1992), for example, noted that individuals satisfying diagnostic criteria for PTSD often scored in the clinical range on a variety of MCMI scales. The reverse also appeared to be true: Individuals with PTSD were likely to appear to have other psychiatric disorders on the MCMI by virtue of the relevance of other scale items to posttraumatic symptomatology.

In contrast to earlier versions of the MCMI, a posttraumatic stress scale (the R scale, in the Clinical Syndromes group) appears in the MCMI-III and the MCMI-IV. However, the content domain of this scale is somewhat problematic. Review of the R scale reveals a majority of items that are not specific to the *DSM-5* diagnostic criteria for PTSD. These include items evaluating sadness, worthlessness, having "strange" thoughts, rapid mood changes, repeated thoughts (content unstated), fears about the future, emptiness, and suicidality. In fact, only 7 of 16 R scale items actually refer to current PTSD criteria: 4 address reexperiencing symptoms, 2 refer to hyperarousal, and 1 taps avoidance. As a result, this scale tends to overvalue reexperiencing phenomena and substantially underestimates avoidance and hyperarousal.

The base rate (BR) standardization method used by the MCMI-III and the MCMI-IV may be affected by the contamination of the R scale with nontrauma-related (primarily depressive) items and its overrepresentation of reexperiencing symptoms. To the extent that these items do not represent the entire (or specific) content domain of PTSD, the MCMI's use of cutting scores to define the presence (BR > 75) or prominence (BR > 85) of PTSD is of questionable merit. Grove and Vrieze (2009) published a critique of the way BRs are calculated on the MCMI-III and proposed solutions that could be considered in the assessment of trauma-related diagnoses. Early research on the MCMI-IV (Mohammadi et al., 2023) showed low diagnostic validity when it comes to PTSD, with sensitivity of 45%, specificity of 82%, and positive predictive probability of only 6.67% based on a Structured Clinical Interview for *DSM-5* (SCID-5) diagnosis. With these results, it can be misleading to state that an individual "has" PTSD by virtue of their MCMI R score, regardless of its BR elevation. Of note, the BR method has also been criticized for unfounded gender differences on the personality scales (specifically on the MCMI-III) once raw scores are transformed into BRs (see Hynan, 2004).

These various concerns do not mean that the R scale is without merit. Rather, the fact that this scale was developed specifically to tap PTSD symptoms (as opposed to the MMPI-2 scales that used existing items and the MMPI-2-RF/MMPI-3 ARX that was designed to measure anxiety symptoms more generally) raises expectations that are only partially met. Ultimately, it may be that the R scale and the MMPI-2 PK scales are, to some extent, measures of a broader, nonspecific range of posttraumatic states rather than of the *DSM-5* diagnostic construct of PTSD per se; and thus, they may reflect more the sequelae of sustained or multievent stressors, wherein depression and related difficulties are especially relevant.

Through use of the PTSD (R) scale, issues associated with misidentification of child abuse survivors and other trauma victims on the MCMI can be reduced. To the extent that the R scale operates as advertised, it can facilitate the interpretation of abuse survivors' MCMI scores by indicating the presence of posttraumatic stress. In such instances, although other less relevant scales (e.g., Thought Disorder) might also be elevated, the presence of a high PTSD score would alert the examiner to the possibility of alternate explanations for such scale elevations. The few studies using the MCMI-III in trauma survivors suggest that the R scale is, in fact, moderately associated with PTSD and other posttraumatic responses (e.g., J. G. Allen et al., 1999; R. J. Craig & Olson, 1997; Hyer et al., 1997). To date, there do not appear to be any studies using the MCMI-IV specifically with a sample of trauma survivors.

Despite its potential limitations, the MCMI-III and MCMI-IV's broad coverage of clinical and personality psychopathology, plus their inclusion of a PTSD-related scale, strengthens their application with trauma survivors— especially in instances in which posttraumatic states coexist with maladaptive personality traits, or where complex PTSD is a possible diagnostic issue. On such occasions, however, the clinician may choose to interpret MCMI results using more accurate statements about personality styles, coping patterns, or psychological defenses, as opposed to diagnosing "personality disorders." Furthermore, clinical experience suggests that the MCMI is a particularly useful tool for informing treatment approaches, which is likely of benefit for more complex cases and individuals with comorbidities as well as trauma effects.

PSYCHOLOGICAL ASSESSMENT INVENTORY

The 344-item Psychological Assessment Inventory (PAI; Morey, 1991, 2007) consists of 22 total scales: 4 validity scales, 11 clinical scales (most of which have scorable subscales), 5 treatment consideration scales, and 2 interpersonal scales. The PAI contains a traumatic stress subscale (Anxiety-Related Disorders– Trauma [ARD-T]), assesses a wide range of symptom presentations, and has superior psychometric characteristics (Morey, 1996). It has been normed on both clinical and community populations.

There is good support for the validity indices on the PAI both in overall profile validity and in the detection of feigned versus genuine PTSD. Specifically, the Negative Distortion scale distinguishes well between individuals with diagnosed PTSD and those instructed to feign PTSD (D. N. Russell & Morey, 2019; K. M. Thomas et al., 2012). One exception is the Negative Impression Management scale, which has been shown to overclassify respondents with dissociative symptoms as exaggerating them (Stadnik et al., 2013). Overall, the PAI validity indices are commonly used symptom validity tests, second only to the MMPI scales (Hawes & Boccaccini, 2009; P. K. Martin et al., 2015).

The ARD-T is one of three components of the full Anxiety-Related Disorders (ARD) scale on the PAI. Five items on the ARD-T tap reexperiencing phenomena, and three are concerned with guilt, loss of interest, and avoidance of memory-triggering stimuli, respectively. Although the ARD-T tends to prioritize posttraumatic reexperiencing over other PTSD symptom clusters, it has shown good diagnostic utility with respect to PTSD (Bellet et al., 2018; McDevitt-Murphy et al., 2007).

Despite its shorter history compared with the MMPI and MCMI scales, research over the past few decades has strongly supported the use of the PAI in PTSD assessment. Specifically, the PAI has identified posttraumatic outcomes and clinically useful profiles in veterans with combat-related PTSD (Ingram et al., 2021; Mozley et al., 2005), motor vehicle accident victims (Holmes et al., 2001), community samples of women (Drury et al., 2009; McDevitt-Murphy et al., 2005), and trauma-exposed college students (McDevitt-Murphy et al., 2007). Next to the ARD-T subscale and the ARD main scale, the most common elevations appear to be on the Depression (DEP), Somatic Complaints (SOM), Anxiety (ANX), Schizophrenia (SCZ), and Borderline Features (BOR) scales (Drury et al., 2009; Holmes et al., 2001; McDevitt-Murphy et al., 2005; Morey, 1996; Mozley et al., 2005). Comorbidity and more complex presentations have been associated with higher scale elevations and a broader range of symptom endorsement (Drury et al., 2009; Mozley et al., 2005).

SYMPTOM CHECKLIST-90-REVISED

The Symptom Checklist-90–Revised (SCL-90-R; Derogatis, 1994) is a widely used self-report measure, based on the earlier Hopkins Symptom Checklist (Derogatis et al., 1974). Derogatis (1993) has since developed the Brief Symptom Inventory, a shorter version of the SCL-90-R. The full measure consists of nine subscales as well as three global indices, including the Global Severity Index. The SCL-90-R has demonstrated high internal consistency and test-retest reliability in clinical as well as nonclinical samples. There are four normative reference groups that can be used for score comparisons: psychiatric outpatients, psychiatric inpatients, nonpatients (a stratified random eastern U.S. sample), and nonpatient adolescents.

The various subscales of the SCL-90-R appear to predict trauma-related disturbance in a wide variety of individuals, including disaster victims (Najarian et al., 2001), Holocaust survivors (Yehuda et al., 1994), rape survivors (Riggs et al., 1992), war veterans (e.g., J. Wolfe et al., 1992), and adults with a history of childhood maltreatment (Gold et al., 1999; Prachason et al., 2024). However, the SCL-90-R does not have a specific scale to assess posttraumatic disturbance, and there is a chance that trauma-related symptoms may be identified by items on other subscales and misinterpreted as obsessive-compulsive, hostile, or psychotic symptomatology, for example. One recent study showed that of the nine SCL-90-R domains, childhood maltreatment exposure explained the most amount of variance in the psychoticism sub-scale in a general population sample of adults (Prachason et al., 2024). It has also been recommended that the SCL-90-R be used primarily as a measure of general psychological distress, given some limitations in the scale's ability to discriminate between specific diagnoses (Hildenbrand et al., 2015).

Although the SCL-90-R does not have a posttraumatic stress scale, researchers have developed new subscales post hoc to assess posttraumatic stress using existing items. One of the more commonly used of these scales was developed by B. E. Saunders and colleagues (1990) and is often referred to as the Crime-Related PTSD scale (CR-PTSD). The CR-PTSD consists of the 28 SCL-90-R items that best discriminated PTSD status in a sample of 355 research participants from the general population. The resultant scale was internally consistent ($\alpha = .93$) and was able to discriminate crime-related PTSD in 89% of cases. Similar results were found in a study with female crime victims (Arata et al., 1991). Subsequently, the psychometric properties of this subscale were examined in two larger college samples (Carlozzi & Long, 2008), further supporting the reliability and validity of the CR-PTSD as a unidimensional measure of posttraumatic stress and as a tool that can discriminate between respondents with and without a PTSD diagnosis.

A second post hoc scale, the War-Zone PTSD scale (WZ-PTSD; F. W. Weathers et al., 1996) is composed of the 25 items on the SCL-90-R that best discriminated 202 Vietnam theater veterans with and without PTSD. The WZ-PTSD scale appears to have very good internal consistency ($\alpha = .97$) and good diagnostic utility with reference to the SCID (Spitzer et al., 1990) or the Clinician-Administered Posttraumatic Stress Disorder Scale (CAPS-1; Blake et al., 1990). Different WZ-PTSD cutoff scores are suggested for the determination of PTSD, based on whether sensitivity (identifying individuals with PTSD) or specificity (identifying individuals without PTSD) is of greater priority.

THE RORSCHACH

The Rorschach projective, or performance-based, test (Rorschach, 1981) consists of 10 bilaterally symmetrical inkblots that are presented to an individual, one at a time. Respondents describe what each inkblot might represent, and their responses are interpreted using one of several systems. For many years, Exner's Comprehensive System (CS; Exner, 2003; Exner et al., 2022) was the most commonly used of these interpretation systems, both clinically and in research. In 2011, the Rorschach Performance Assessment System (R-PAS; Meyer et al., 2011) was released by members of Exner's Rorschach Research Council. The R-PAS is empirically based, is internationally normed, and is reportedly easier to use than Exner's CS. As is true of the other standard measures reviewed here, the Rorschach has some advantages and disadvantages in the assessment of posttraumatic states. On one hand, it provides an opportunity to assess phenomena beyond the capacities of objective testing wherein the client is forced to respond to a specific test item and therefore to a specific mini-hypothesis regarding the structure of psychological disturbance. Instead, the Rorschach offers a set of relatively ambiguous stimuli, to which the client may respond in any manner they choose. As a result, the client's responses are less predetermined and potentially freer to accurately reflect whatever trauma effects might be discoverable. It is also theorized that some respondents might be better able to access their trauma-related beliefs and internal experiences when they do not have to report directly on details of the trauma itself (Luxenberg & Levin, 2004). On the other hand, the interpretation systems used to classify Rorschach responses are not entirely free of theoretical assumptions, and they can introduce a level of misinterpretation when posttraumatic symptomatology is present. Overall, opinions range on the validity of the Rorschach in standard clinical assessment. Some point out that it has a similar level of validity to the MMPI (.30; Groth-Marnat, 2003; Viglione et al., 2012) and that it potentially adds incremental information (Luxenberg & Levin, 2004), whereas others believe it is too labor-intensive and of limited reliability (Wood et al., 2003). Use of the Rorschach in forensic assessments is controversial and generally cautioned against (for review, see Viglione et al., 2022).

Use of the Rorschach to Assess Posttraumatic States

Viglione and colleagues (2012) provided a detailed summary of how to use the Rorschach when assessing posttraumatic states. They suggested five areas in which the Rorschach can provide valuable information: (a) cognitive constriction, (b) trauma-related imagery, (c) trauma-related cognitive disturbances, (d) stress response, and (e) dissociation. They emphasized that the Rorschach should not be used as a diagnostic measure of PTSD; rather, "the test may function better as a description of the impact and possible forms that trauma may take in the respondent's life" (p. 142). To that end, the indicators discussed next may provide informative contributions to an assessment of posttraumatic states and experiences. For more detailed information on the use of the Rorschach in trauma-related assessment, see Viglione et al. (2012) and Luxenberg and Levin (2004).

The Traumatic Content Index (TC/R) may be the most obvious indicator of trauma-related disturbance on the Rorschach. The TC/R was created by Armstrong and Loewenstein (1990), who defined it as "the sum of the sex, blood, and anatomy content scores plus the morbid and aggressive special scores divided by the total number of responses" (p. 450) and expressed it as a percentage. Understandably, this captures some, but not all, content related to trauma exposure and triggered memories. In at least one study (Kamphuis et al., 2000), the TC/R distinguished between women with and without documented sexual abuse histories.

Other CS scoring indicators that might provide information about a respondent's posttraumatic symptoms and experiences include a low affective ratio (Afr), a high Hypervigilance Index (HVI), and a low D (Common Detail Response) or high adjusted D (AdjD) score. Specifically, a low Afr is a measure of affect avoidance, especially in combination with an elevated Lambda (L), and is thought to approximate numbing and avoidance symptoms seen in PTSD sufferers (Armstrong & Kaser-Boyd, 2004; Hartman et al., 1990; Kaser-Boyd, 1993). A high HVI was originally thought to identify paranoia but this can also be an indicator of hyperarousal or vigilance to trauma-related threats often associated with PTSD (Luxenberg & Levin, 2004). Finally, low D scores, such as those found in veterans with diagnosed PTSD (Weiner, 1996), are a possible indication that an individual's attempts to cope are undermined by chronic intrusions and a sense of helplessness.

A significant risk of using the Rorschach when assessing posttraumatic states is the very real possibility that trauma-related presentations can be misinterpreted as evidence of a psychotic or personality disorder (e.g., Luxenberg & Levin, 2004; E. A. Saunders, 1991). For example, in an early Rorschach study of war veterans, those with PTSD seemingly revealed signs of thought disorder or impaired reality testing (van der Kolk & Ducey, 1984, 1989). The potential overlap between psychotic, personality-disordered, and posttraumatic Rorschach presentations requires the clinician to be familiar with all three diagnostic scenarios and their Rorschach representations when evaluating posttraumatic dysfunction or disorder. Results that are suggestive of a psychotic disorder, such as a positive Schizophrenia Index, should be carefully considered in a respondent who does not show any signs of psychosis in everyday life but does have a trauma history. Finally, these indicators offer very little discrimination between types of posttraumatic disturbance. For example, although a given study may find that clients with dissociative disorder score higher on unstructured color or morbid content relative to norms, it is not clear whether this difference represents dissociation, differences in clinical acuity between samples, comorbid posttraumatic stress, or perhaps the generalized effects of a trauma history on emotional regulation capacities. For this reason, the clinician is advised to use caution in making especially specific interpretations regarding what otherwise might be more general posttraumatic Rorschach responses.

CONCLUSION

Traditional objective and projective psychological tests can be an important part of the trauma-focused assessment battery. First, generic tests provide important information on comorbid phenomena, such as the presence of anxiety, depression, personality disorder, or psychosis. Second, when trauma-specific scales or scoring procedures are available, such instruments may signal the presence of posttraumatic disturbance. Finally, in most cases, these scales are normed on general population samples, allowing the clinician to interpret specific scores in terms of their extremity, if not severity.

Unfortunately, almost none of the currently available generic measures, with or without trauma-specific features, are especially sensitive to posttraumatic stress. These measures typically include a variety of items that are not directly related to posttraumatic symptomatology, do not well represent the four symptom clusters of PTSD, and do not assess symptoms within the 1-month timeframe required by the *DSM-5*. Equally important, almost none of these measures test for acute stress disorder or dissociative disorders. As a result, it is recommended that generic tests either be administered or followed up with more specialized trauma measures whenever possible, rather than being used in isolation to index posttraumatic disturbance.

7 TRAUMA-SPECIFIC TESTS

In addition to the generic psychological tests outlined in Chapter 6 of this volume, there are a number of trauma-specific objective measures available to clinicians. These measures usually approach posttraumatic difficulties from one of the following perspectives:

- diagnostic, criterion-based measures that tend to focus on *Diagnostic and Statistical Manual of Mental Disorders* (*DSM*) diagnoses (although some also measure symptom severity);

- instruments that assess a range of posttraumatic symptomatology, including presentations more relevant to complex posttraumatic stress disorder (PTSD); and

- more specific tools that measure a component of posttraumatic disturbance other than, but often related to, PTSD (e.g., dissociation, posttraumatic cognitions, traumatic grief).

There are strengths and weaknesses associated with trauma-specific objective measures. Advantages include (a) avoidance of the subjectivity sometimes associated with diagnostic interviews (trauma-based or otherwise) and the ability of individuals to report on their own experiences; (b) the reliability

https://doi.org/10.1037/0000452-007
Psychological Assessment of Adult Posttraumatic States: Phenomenology, Diagnosis, and Measurement, Third Edition, by E. M. Eadie and J. Briere

they offer, by virtue of multiple items addressing the same or related phenomena; (c) the reduced need for trained and qualified clinicians to be physically present during parts of the evaluation; and (d) the ease with which such tests can be administered, both in terms of the amount of time involved per test and the possibility of assessing multiple individuals simultaneously.

There are also drawbacks of trauma-specific self-report measures that the clinician should keep in mind. First, research clinicians have tended to produce slightly different versions of essentially the same trauma measure, at least with reference to PTSD. During the era of the *DSM*'s revised third and fourth editions (*DSM-III-R* & *DSM-IV*; American Psychiatric Association, 1987, 1994), numerous self-report measures were created consisting of what were then the 17 symptoms of PTSD (Carlson, 1997). Many of these measures have been updated to 20 items as the diagnostic criteria have expanded with the fifth edition (*DSM-5*; American Psychiatric Association, 2013), but others have become outdated. These measures differ primarily in terms of how symptoms are worded using lay language, with most differences in reliability and validity associated with the degree of success with this endeavor and the samples used to validate each measure. Not only is this approach somewhat redundant, but it also creates inherent limitations in the resultant instruments. For example, in most cases, such measures provide only one item per PTSD symptom. If the subject misinterprets or avoids that item, the underlying construct goes unassessed or is distorted. Furthermore, according to standard measurement theory, a single item is often a less reliable estimate of a construct than are several items—leading to error variation in the assessment of flashbacks or psychic numbing, for example.

Second, most PTSD measures examine only the four symptom clusters represented in the *DSM-5* and its text revision (*DSM-5-TR*; American Psychiatric Association, 2022; i.e., posttraumatic reexperiencing, avoidance, negative cognitions and mood, and hyperarousal) or the three symptom clusters described in the *DSM-IV* (i.e., reexperiencing, avoidance, and hyperarousal). Yet, as outlined in Chapter 2 and elsewhere in this volume, posttraumatic stress may include a variety of other comorbid states or responses, including dissociation, somatization, attachment and interpersonal difficulties, and disturbance in self-organization (DSOs). Although sometimes all that is needed is a brief PTSD screen, in many cases a comprehensive trauma assessment may be more appropriate, such as examining the presence of DSOs and dissociation as well as more classic notions of posttraumatic stress.

Third, as noted in Chapter 6, objective measures that use a total score to reflect posttraumatic stress inappropriately collapse all PTSD dimensions into a single number. Although total scores can be helpful for monitoring progress in treatment or getting a quick, overall view of severity level, a disadvantage exists in the loss of information. On any given instrument, there may be several different ways for respondents to achieve the same total score: For one respondent, one score may represent a broad spread of moderate endorsement across most or all symptoms; for another respondent, the same score might represent high endorsement of only one or two symptom clusters. Clearly, these different responses represent different clinical scenarios, each of which should ideally be evaluated with separate scales.

Finally, although a number of trauma-specific measures demonstrate reliability and validity in research contexts, fewer are developed to the point where they can be used unambiguously in clinical settings. Most importantly, many of these instruments are not accompanied by appropriate normative data. As a result, the clinician has almost no way of determining to what extent, if at all, the respondent's level of symptom endorsement is greater than what most people would endorse. In contrast, standardized measures allow the evaluator to compare the client's score with that of the general population and determine how deviant (i.e., clinically significant) it is. In the case of instruments whose sole purpose is diagnostic screening, the absence of normative data generally is less of a problem, because the issue of concern is whether a given set of symptoms are (or are not) present. For continuous measures of a clinical construct, however, the evaluator is left not knowing whether a given score is normal or symptomatic. On occasion, this problem is partially addressed by cutting scores, wherein any score at or above a particular value is reported to be associated with a given diagnosis with a certain level of probability. However, the appropriate cutoff may vary from sample to sample, and this approach does not allow for interpretation of the entire range of scores below (or even above) the cut point.

Because of these concerns, the clinician is advised to limit their interpretation of scores on nonstandardized trauma-specific measures. In some cases, the best the examiner may be able to say is that approximately $X\%$ of research participants with Y disorder scored higher or lower than the respondent (based on available means and standard deviations) in a given sample in a given published study. In such cases, the examiner should also describe the extent to which the respondent matches the demographics and clinical status of that sample.

SCREENING TOOLS

In many settings, it is useful to begin an assessment with a brief measure that screens for the likely presence of PTSD. The screening tools listed next are, for the most part, very short (ranging from 4 to 14 items) and quick to administer, making them efficient for use in settings where time is limited or there is a need to identify those who would benefit most from a longer, more comprehensive diagnostic assessment. However, the information provided by these screeners is partial and limited in scope. Accordingly, these tools should not be used, on their own, to make diagnostic or treatment decisions. Instead, any positive screen is an indication that the assessor should proceed with a more detailed and systematic assessment covering the full range of diagnostic indicators for PTSD as well as potential differential diagnoses.

Primary Care PTSD Screen for *DSM-5*

The five-item Primary Care PTSD Screen for *DSM-5* (PC-PTSD-5; Prins et al., 2015) was developed to screen for PTSD in primary care settings. At the outset, respondents are asked about lifetime trauma exposure; if they report such exposure, they proceed to answer five dichotomously scored (*yes* or *no*) questions about how that exposure has affected them over the past month.

Based on research with a large sample of U.S. Department of Veterans Affairs primary care patients, Bovin and colleagues (2021) recommended a PC-PTSD-5 cutoff score of 4 (i.e., endorsement of four of five items) to identify those who screened positive for probable PTSD. In their study, this score balanced false-negative and false-positive results with respect to the overall sample and male participants. However, for women, a threshold score of 4 produced a higher proportion of false-negative results. Consequently, the authors recommended that a cut point of 3 may be more suitable when using the PC-PTSD-5 with women (Bovin et al., 2021).

PTSD and Suicide Screener

The brief, 14-item self-report PTSD and Suicide Screener (PSS; Briere, 2013) was derived using items from the Detailed Assessment of Posttraumatic Stress (DAPS; Briere, 2001).[1] The PSS consists of two scales: PTSD Risk (PR; eight items) and Suicide Risk (SR; four items), with items rated on a 5-point scale (1 = *never* to 5 = *four or more times a week*). The PR scale contains items that tap all symptom clusters from both *DSM-IV* and *DSM-5*

---

[1]It should be noted that one of the authors of this book (J. Briere) has developed a number of the trauma-relevant tests described here and elsewhere. The reader should keep this proprietary connection in mind when considering the information presented. That said, the authors have endeavored to evaluate all tests objectively, and evaluations of his tests were written by the first author (E. M. Eadie).

diagnostic criteria. Risk indices are based on cutoff scores that were empirically derived from two normative samples. Both the PR and SR scales are internally consistent (α = .87 and .91, respectively), and the PR scale has good sensitivity and specificity for a diagnosis of PTSD from the text revision of the *DSM-IV* (*DSM-IV-TR*; American Psychiatric Association, 2000).

Screen for Posttraumatic Stress Symptoms

The Screen for Posttraumatic Stress Symptoms (SPTSS; Carlson, 2001) was developed as a PTSD screening measure. In contrast to many other brief instruments, this test does not assess symptoms associated with a single traumatic event, making it an especially useful tool for individuals with multiple traumatic events or an unknown trauma history. The SPTSS inquires about any PTSD-related symptoms experienced by the respondent over the past 2 weeks. Items are rated from 0 (*never*) to 10 (*always*). An alternative version is available with a 5-point rating scale from 0 (*not at all*) to 4 (*more than once a day*).

The SPTSS total score is internally consistent, yielding an α of .91 in a sample of 136 psychiatric inpatients (Carlson, 2001). In addition, the total scale score correlates as expected with other brief trauma impact measures. Using the recommended cutoff of 4, the SPTSS had a sensitivity of .94 and a specificity of .60 in the prediction of PTSD. Although other cutoffs would have yielded a different balance of sensitivity and specificity, Carlson chose this score to maximize the likelihood that the SPTSS would identify most actual cases of PTSD in clinical groups. The low specificity of this score, of course, means that some patients without PTSD will be identified as potentially screening positive for PTSD, reinforcing that this tool should only be used for screening and not diagnostic purposes.

Short Posttraumatic Stress Disorder Rating Interview

The eight-item Short Posttraumatic Stress Disorder Rating Interview (SPRINT; Connor & Davidson, 2001) assesses the severity of posttraumatic stress symptoms whether or not the respondent meets diagnostic criteria for PTSD. The items assess the four domains of PTSD (intrusion, avoidance, numbing, and arousal) as well as somatic complaints, vulnerability to stress, and functional impairment. Symptoms are rated from 0 (*not at all*) to 4 (*very much*), and two additional items ask for the respondent's subjective rating of treatment response. The authors recommended a cutoff score of 14 and noted that scores of 18 or above would correspond to severe posttraumatic stress.

The SPRINT has good internal consistency (α = .88), high test-retest reliability (intraclass correlation coefficient = .78), and strong convergent and divergent validity and it is sensitive to treatment effects. It has also been shown to correlate well with the Clinician-Administered PTSD Scale (CAPS; Vaishnavi et al., 2006). The SPRINT was not intended to correspond to a specific *DSM* edition and has not been updated for the *DSM-5*.

SPAN Self-Report Screen

The four-item SPAN (Davidson, 2002) self-report screen assesses the following symptoms: Startle, Physiological arousal, Anger, and Numbness. The items are derived from the Davidson Trauma Scale (DTS) and best distinguish individuals with PTSD from those without. Items are rated from 0 (*not at all distressing*) to 4 (*extremely distressing*) over the past week. A total score of 5 or more is considered a positive screen. The SPAN has good convergent validity, a sensitivity of .84, and a specificity of .91. Its diagnostic accuracy is 88% and it has been shown to be responsive to treatment effects (Meltzer-Brody et al., 1999).

STANDARDIZED ASSESSMENT SCALES AND DIAGNOSTIC TOOLS

There are several measures that, by virtue of their standardization, their psychometric qualities, and, in most cases, their normative data, are appropriate for general use in clinical settings. A few additional scales are included here because although they are not normed, they are helpful in gathering criterion-based information to support diagnoses.

Measures of Posttraumatic Stress and Acute Stress

The following instruments gather information about symptoms of PTSD and acute stress disorder (ASD) and are among the most commonly used scales in the assessment of traumatic stress.

Acute Stress Disorder Scale-5

The self-report Acute Stress Disorder Scale (ASDS; Bryant, 2016; Bryant et al., 2000) was developed to assist in the diagnosis of ASD and to predict later PTSD. It assesses 14 symptoms of traumatic stress in the acute period after trauma exposure (i.e., 3 days to 1 month). The ASDS was developed originally to meet *DSM-IV* ASD criteria (Bryant et al., 2000) and has been updated to correspond to *DSM-5* criteria (ASDS-5; Bryant, 2016).

Although psychometric data on the updated ASDS-5 are not yet available, the prior version was validated by Bryant and colleagues (2000), who found high internal consistency (total score $\alpha = .96$) and test-retest reliability

($r = .94$) across 2 to 7 days. The ASDS reexperiencing, avoidance, and hyper-arousal scale scores correlated as expected with equivalent scale scores on the Impact of Events Scale and the Beck Anxiety Inventory (Beck & Steer, 1993), although the ASDS dissociation score did not correlate with the taxon score of the Dissociative Experiences Scale (DES-T; Waller et al., 1996). The ASDS has a sensitivity of .95 and a specificity of .83 vis-à-vis a diagnosis of ASD on the Acute Stress Disorder Structured Interview (ASDI). Although this is a very good result, the authors acknowledged that the items of the ASDS were modeled specifically on those of the ASDI and "therefore we would expect strong convergence between these two indexes" (Bryant et al., 2000, p. 65).

Davidson Trauma Scale

The 17-item DTS (Davidson, Book, et al., 1997) measures *DSM-IV* PTSD criteria on 5-point frequency ($0 = not\ at\ all$ to $4 = every\ day$) and severity ($0 = not\ at\ all\ distressing$ to $4 = extremely\ distressing$) scales over the past week. Respondents anchor their symptom ratings to a specific index trauma. This measure yields a total score, as well as scale scores for Intrusion, Avoidance/Numbing, and Hyperarousal. Because the DTS is used primarily to render a probable diagnosis of PTSD, there are no associated normative data for interpreting test scores.

The DTS has good test-retest reliability ($r = .86$) and internal consistency (α ranging from .97 to .99), as well as concurrent validity. Criterion validity has been assessed with reference to the SCID, in which a score of 40 on the DTS had a sensitivity of .69 and a specificity of .95. Although this agreement with positive SCID PTSD cases is less than stellar, the high specificity supports its use as a conservative measure of posttraumatic stress. In a subsequent study, Davidson and colleagues (2002) found that the sensitivity of the DTS in detecting effects of medication (selective serotonin reuptake inhibitors) on posttraumatic stress was equal to, or better than, that found for three other trauma measures, including the CAPS. As noted earlier, the SPAN Self-Report Screen (Davidson, 2002) is derived from items in the DTS.

Detailed Assessment of Posttraumatic Stress

The comprehensive 104-item DAPS inventory (Briere, 2001) provides information on an adult client's history of trauma exposure (Trauma Specification and Relative Trauma Exposure). The DAPS also includes scales that assess the following: immediate cognitive, emotional, and dissociative reactions (Peritraumatic Distress and Peritraumatic Dissociation); subsequent posttraumatic stress symptoms (Reexperiencing, Avoidance, and Hyperarousal); and associated impact on functioning (Posttraumatic Impairment) in the context of a specific traumatic event. In addition to a narrative report, the DAPS interpretive program (Briere et al., 2003) provides additional information on the Avoidance scale, yielding separate scores for the Effortful Avoidance and Numbing symptom clusters. This measure has two validity scales that evaluate under- and overreport of symptoms (Positive Bias and Negative Bias, respectively), and three scales that measure common PTSD-related comorbidities (Trauma-Specific Dissociation, Substance Abuse, and Suicidality). Like the Posttraumatic Stress Diagnostic Scale (PDS) and the DTS, the DAPS provides a potential *DSM-IV* diagnosis of PTSD. In addition, it yields a tentative diagnosis of *DSM-IV* ASD. An updated version (DAPS-2) is in progress at the time of this writing, which will provide a provisional *DSM-5* diagnosis (see Petri et al., 2020).

The DAPS was normed on a sample of 433 adults in the general population who had experienced at least one *DSM-IV* Criterion A traumatic event. The scales of this instrument are internally consistent, with an average α of .82 on the clinical scales. In the validation sample, DAPS scales tapping posttraumatic stress symptoms (Reexperiencing, Avoidance, and Hyperarousal) were strongly associated with other measures of the same constructs (e.g., the Impact of Events Scale [IES] and relevant scales of the CAPS). The associated features scales of the DAPS demonstrate evidence of discriminant validity: The DAPS Peritraumatic Dissociation scale correlates highest with the Peritraumatic Dissociative Experiences Questionnaire (PDEQ; Marmar et al., 1997), the Trauma-Specific Dissociation scale is most related to the Multiscale Dissociation Inventory (MDI; Briere, 2002) total score, Substance Abuse has the highest correlation with the PAI Alcohol and Drug scales, and Suicidality is most associated with the PAI Suicidal Ideation scale. The DAPS has good sensitivity (.88) and specificity (.86) in detecting PTSD status on the CAPS, with an associated κ of .73.

Global Psychotrauma Screen

The 22-item self-report Global Psychotrauma Screen (GPS; Olff et al., 2020) was developed by the Global Collaboration on Traumatic Stress. The GPS begins by identifying an index trauma and then asks about the presence (*yes* or *no*) of symptoms occurring in the past month. Items do not map directly onto *DSM-5* criteria but instead include a range of posttraumatic symptoms, such as sleep difficulties, self-injurious behavior, dissociation, and substance use, in addition to symptoms of intrusion, avoidance, and hypervigilance. Additional items ask about risk and protective factors thought to influence the course of posttraumatic symptoms. The GPS can be completed in paper-and-pencil form, on the website, or through an app, with the latter two options providing direct feedback to the respondent. The GPS is available in 27 languages and normative data are available from several countries, making this one of the more internationally accessible tools. The authors reported good preliminary reliability and concurrent validity across multiple samples from different countries.

Posttraumatic Stress Checklist for *DSM-5*
The Posttraumatic Stress Checklist for *DSM-5* (PCL-5; F. W. Weathers, Litz, et al., 2013) is one of the most widely used self-report scales for posttraumatic stress symptoms. The 20-item PCL-5 is an updated version of the previous Posttraumatic Stress Disorder Checklist (PCL; Weathers et al., 1993), and it can be used to monitor symptoms over time and to assist in making a provisional diagnosis of PTSD. Items are rated on a 5-point scale from 0 (*not at all*) to 4 (*extremely*). Different versions allow for symptoms to be measured over two different time frames: past week or past month. The PCL-5 is often administered alongside the Life Events Checklist for *DSM-5* for assessment of trauma history. If multiple traumatic events are identified, the respondent is instructed to base their symptom responses on the "worst event." A total severity score, as well as scores for each of the *DSM-5* diagnostic clusters (i.e., reexperiencing, avoidance, negative cognitions and mood, and hyperarousal), can be generated.

Although a provisional PTSD diagnosis can be made using cluster scores and following the *DSM-5* diagnostic algorithm, F. W. Weathers, Litz, and colleagues (2013) stated that a total severity score in the range of 31 to 33 is an indication of probable PTSD. The PCL-5 has good psychometric qualities, with high internal consistency ($\alpha = .94$ to .96), good test-retest reliability ($r = .74$ to .85), and good convergent and discriminant validity. It is relatively sensitive to change over time, making it a useful measure to assess treatment progress (Blevins et al., 2015; Bovin et al., 2016).

Posttraumatic Stress Diagnostic Scale
The PDS-5 (Foa et al., 2016a) is an updated version of the original PDS (Foa, 1995). The scale begins with two screening questions to assess trauma history and to identify a specific index trauma. It consists of 24 items assessing each of the *DSM-5* PTSD symptoms, as well as 2 items examining level of distress and interference caused by the symptoms and 2 items measuring onset and duration of symptoms. Items are rated on a combined frequency and severity scale from 0 (*not at all*) to 4 (*6 or more times a week/severe*).

The PDS-5 has excellent internal consistency ($\alpha = .95$), excellent test-retest reliability ($r = .90$), and good convergent and discriminant validity. There was 78% agreement between the PDS-5 and the PSSI-5, the semistructured interview by the same authors. A cutoff score of 28 is recommended for identification of probable PTSD diagnosis (Foa et al., 2016a).

Dissociation Measures

Although dissociation is an important component of posttraumatic response, the majority of clinical assessment in this area has employed the Dissociative Experiences Scale (DES-II). The DES-II, along with other dissociation measures, is described in the "Nonstandardized Assessment Tools" section in this chapter. The only standardized and normed measure of dissociation, the MDI, is presented here.

Multiscale Dissociation Inventory

The 30-item MDI (Briere, 2002) is a test of dissociative symptomatology. Based on research suggesting that dissociation is a multidimensional phenomenon, the MDI (Briere, 2002) consists of six scales (Disengagement, Depersonalization, Derealization, Memory Disturbance, Emotional Constriction, and Identity Dissociation). Each symptom is rated according to its frequency of occurrence over the previous month on a scale ranging from 1 (*never*) to 5 (*very often*). The MDI was normed on 444 trauma-exposed individuals from the general population. Scale scores can be converted to *T*-scores that allow for empirically based clinical interpretation of clients' level of dissociative disturbance. Because the different forms of dissociation are measured separately on the MDI, a score profile is generated for each client, rather than the single dissociation score generated by some other measures.

The MDI had good psychometric qualities in normative and validation samples. Differential relationships were found between MDI scales and demographics, trauma history, posttraumatic stress, measures of attention and processing speed, and scores on other dissociation measures (e.g., Briere, 2002; Dietrich, 2003; Parlar et al., 2016). Furthermore, a raw score of 15 or higher on the MDI Identity Dissociation scale identified 93% of individuals with diagnosis of dissociative identity disorder (DID)[2] and 92% of those with no diagnosis of DID in a combined clinical/community sample (Briere, 2002).

Measures of Complex Posttraumatic Stress Disorder and Disturbances in Self-Organization

As noted in Chapter 2, early and chronic psychological trauma can result in DSOs (Bachem et al., 2021), involving impaired self-concept, relational functioning, and emotional regulation. DSOs are a component of the *International Classification of Diseases, Eleventh Revision (ICD-11*; World Health

---

[2]In all but two instances, diagnosis was based on the SCID-D.

Organization, 2022) diagnostic criteria for complex PTSD. In addition to the tools described here, the Trauma Symptom Inventory–2 (TSI-2), discussed in this section, has two scales (Impaired Self-Reference and Tension Reduction Behavior) that tap identity and emotion regulation symptoms.

Bell Object Relations and Reality Testing Inventory

The Bell Object Relations and Reality Testing Inventory (BORRTI; M. D. Bell, 1995) is the only standardized test of what is generally referred to as *disturbed object relations*—a clinical construct that is, in some ways, similar to DSOs. The BORRTI has scales that yield data on four object relations constructs: Alienation, Insecure Attachment, Egocentricity, and Social Incompetence. These scales were shown by the test author to predict and potentially explain relational difficulties in individuals thought to have some form of personality disorder. BORRTI item content also reflects identity issues and affect regulation difficulties, although there are no scales specifically tapping those domains. More recently, convergent and discriminant validity were demonstrated alongside a performance-based measure of object relations (Pad et al., 2020). Because the scales are linked to object relations theory, the results of this measure will be most directly applicable to clinicians who endorse that perspective. A very small literature in this area suggests that the BORRTI may be helpful in evaluating self-organization and attachment issues in traumatized populations (e.g., Alpher, 1991; Haviland et al., 1995; Santina, 1998).

International Trauma Questionnaire

The 18-item self-report International Trauma Questionnaire (ITQ; Cloitre et al., 2018) measures the core features of PTSD and complex PTSD according to the *ICD-11* criteria, although with potentially insufficient coverage of dissociation. Items assess the three *ICD-11* domains of PTSD symptoms: reexperiencing, avoidance, and sense of current threat. The remaining items measure the three DSOs (affective dysregulation, negative self-concept, and disturbances in relationships) that are required to make a diagnosis of complex PTSD. Items on the ITQ are intentionally easy to understand and are rated on a 5-point scale from 0 (*not at all*) to 4 (*extremely*). Respondents are asked to identify an index trauma and base their responses on that experience. Both diagnostic (for *ICD-11* PTSD and complex PTSD) and dimensional scoring rules are available.

The ITQ was validated on a large community sample and a trauma-exposed clinical sample (Cloitre et al., 2018). Research has found the ITQ to have good psychometric qualities, including criterion validity for complex PTSD (Karatzias et al., 2017; Shevlin et al., 2018).

Inventory of Altered Self Capacities

The Inventory of Altered Self Capacities (IASC; Briere, 2000b) is a normed and standardized test of difficulties in the areas of relatedness, identity, and emotional regulation. The IASC scales assess the following domains: Interpersonal Conflicts, Idealization-Disillusionment, Abandonment Concerns, Identity Impairment, Susceptibility to Influence, Affect Dysregulation, and Tension Reduction Activities. Items are rated on a 4-point frequency scale ranging from 1 (*never*) to 4 (*often*) as they occurred over the previous 6 months. The IASC was standardized and normed on 620 general population participants and various clinical and university samples. It was found to be reliable (with an average α across scales of .89) and to have good convergent and discriminant validity in both normative and validation samples. The IASC scales have been shown in a number of studies to predict child maltreatment history, adult attachment style, borderline and antisocial personality features, interpersonal problems, suicidality, dysfunctional sexual behavior, and substance abuse (e.g., B. Allen, 2011; Bigras et al., 2015; Briere & Runtz, 2002). The IASC was also designed to predict certain issues (e.g., abandonment fears and idealization or devaluation) that otherwise might disrupt or derail the client–therapist relationship during treatment.

Trauma Symptom Inventory–2

The 136-item TSI-2 (Briere, 2011), a revision of the TSI, is a standardized test of acute and chronic posttraumatic symptomatology and related concerns. Respondents rate items on a 4-point frequency scale ranging from 0 (*never*) to 3 (*often*) over the previous 6 months. Symptom responses are not specifically linked to an index trauma or adverse event; although the TSI-2 assesses many PTSD symptoms, it also evaluates a broader range of trauma-related concerns.

Normed on a representative sample of the U.S. general population, the TSI-2 has 2 validity scales, 12 clinical scales (with 10 items each), and 4 summary factors validated by confirmatory factor analysis (Godbout et al., 2016). On the posttraumatic stress factor, there are scales assessing Intrusive Experiences, Defensive Avoidance, Dissociation, and Anxious Arousal. On the self-disturbance factor, Insecure Attachment, Impaired Self-Reference, and Depression are examined. The externalizing factor consists of four clinical scales: Anger, Suicidality, Sexual Disturbance, and Tension Reduction Behavior. Finally, the somatization factor taps general somatic symptoms as well as pain-specific concerns. Adding to its clinical utility, the TSI-2 includes eight critical items that identify safety concerns and potentially severe disturbance. It also has *reliable change scores* that can be used for repeat administrations, including treatment progress.

The TSI-2 is reliable and internally consistent (with an average α of .88 on the clinical scales), and it was found to have good convergent and discriminant validity in both normative and validation samples. Its psychometric properties have been replicated in a number of studies (e.g., Filone & DeMatteo, 2017; Nilsson et al., 2018).

Trauma-Related Cognitive Measures

Research has increasingly revealed the importance of posttraumatic cognitions, both as a symptomatic response itself as well as an antecedent to negative emotional states and dysfunctional behavior. Although a number of clinical measures of general cognitive disturbance are available to the clinician, especially with regard to low self-esteem, there are only a few clinical tests of trauma-specific cognitions and beliefs. The two tests that are standardized are discussed here.

Trauma and Attachment Belief Scale

The Trauma and Attachment Belief Scale (TABS; Pearlman, 2003; formerly the Traumatic Stress Institute Belief Scale) is a normed and standardized instrument that measures disrupted cognitive schema and need states associated with trauma exposure. It evaluates beliefs about self and others on five dimensions: Safety, Trust, Esteem, Intimacy, and Control. Items in each domain are rated separately for self and others, generating 10 subscales (e.g., Self-Safety, Other-Safety). Items are rated on a 6-point agreement scale from 1 (*disagree strongly*) to 6 (*agree strongly*).

The TABS has good internal consistency ($\alpha = .96$) and test-retest reliability ($r = .75$). Previous versions of the TABS have been used to measure vicarious traumatization in therapists (e.g., Pearlman & Saakvitne, 1995), as well as to evaluate the effects of trauma on college students, outpatients, survivors of interpersonal violence, and individuals experiencing homelessness (Pearlman, 2003). In contrast to more symptom-based tests, the TABS measures the self-reported needs and expectations of trauma survivors and their perceptions of these phenomena in others. As a result, this measure is helpful in understanding important assumptions that the client carries in their relationships to others, including the therapist, and in formulating more relational (as opposed to solely symptom-focused) treatment goals.

Cognitive Distortions Scale

The 40-item Cognitive Distortions Scale (CDS; Briere, 2000a) measures five types of cognitive symptoms or distortions found among mental health clients and those who have experienced interpersonal victimization, including child abuse: self-criticism, self-blame, helplessness, hopelessness, and preoccupation with danger. Each item is rated according to its frequency of occurrence over the previous month, using a 5-point scale ranging from 1 (*never*) to 5 (*very often*). The CDS scales are internally consistent (with α values ranging from .89 to .97) and demonstrated convergent validity with other cognitive distortion measures in the standardization and validity samples. Validation studies reported in the CDS manual indicate that CDS scales are predictive of interpersonal victimization history, suicidality, depression, and posttraumatic stress. Scales are normed separately for males and females and are expressed as *T*-scores.

NONSTANDARDIZED ASSESSMENT TOOLS

The trauma field has produced several other instruments that measure some aspect of trauma-related concerns but have not yet been fully standardized and normed. Most of these nonstandardized assessment tools have been developed in a research context and may have limited use in clinical practice.

Measures of Posttraumatic Stress and Acute Stress

The majority of nonstandardized posttraumatic stress scales were developed in the 1980s to early 1990s, in response to growing research interest in PTSD. Many of these scales have become outdated as our understanding of PTSD and ASD has grown and the diagnostic criteria have changed. Reviewed next are three nonstandardized scales that remain in frequent use or serve a specific purpose in the assessment landscape.

Impact of Events Scale–Revised

The Impact of Events Scale–Revised (IES-R; Weiss & Marmar, 1997) is an updated version of the IES (Horowitz et al., 1979), one of the earliest self-report measures of posttraumatic disturbance. This 22-item instrument evaluates trauma-related intrusion, avoidance, and hyperarousal symptoms related to a specific stressful life event. Respondents rate symptoms over the past 7 days on a 5-point scale from 0 (*not at all*) to 4 (*extremely*). A total severity score, along with three subscale scores (Intrusion, Avoidance, and Hyperarousal), can be generated. The authors indicated that mean scores should be calculated for the subscales rather than raw sums so these scores can be directly compared to client responses on the Symptom Checklist-90–Revised

(Derogatis, 1994). The IES-R does not cover all of the diagnostic criteria for PTSD, and it has not been updated to correspond with the *DSM-5*.

Psychometric properties of the IES-R were studied in civilian (Weiss & Marmar, 1997) and veteran samples (Creamer et al., 2003). It was found to have high internal consistency and strong convergent validity with the PCL. However, the factor structure was not supported in either study.

Harvard Trauma Questionnaire

The trauma exposure section of the Harvard Trauma Questionnaire (HTQ; Mollica et al., 1992) was described in Chapter 4 (this volume). This measure also has a section to assess both PTSD and non-PTSD symptoms. The PTSD symptom component consists of 16 items that can be scored to indicate a possible *DSM-IV* diagnosis of PTSD. There are also 14 items that evaluate other aspects of culturally specific distress. Although there are relatively few psychometric data available on this measure, the HTQ may be especially useful when examining severe, politically motivated trauma, including torture (Kleijn et al., 2001; Mollica et al., 1992; Smith Fawzi et al., 1997), and when used with refugees or residents of Indochina. When administered to individuals from other cultures and geographic regions, only the 16 PTSD items may be directly applicable as written. In support of cultural adaptation rather than mere language translation, the authors recommended adjusting additional items so they are specific and relevant to the culture of respondents (Mollica et al., 1996).

Stanford Acute Stress Reaction Questionnaire

The Stanford Acute Stress Reaction Questionnaire (SASRQ; Cardeña et al., 1996) was the first measure of ASD symptoms to appear in the traumatic stress literature. Unlike the ASDS-5 (reviewed earlier in this chapter), the SASRQ does not generate a likely diagnosis of ASD; rather, it assesses a range of acute stress reactions, including intrusion, avoidance, arousal, dissociative, and mood-related symptoms, as well as functional impairment, symptom duration, and timing of the trauma exposure. The original validation study demonstrated that the SASRQ is internally consistent and relatively stable across time when no traumas intervene (Cardeña et al., 2000). As expected, this scale also predicts later PTSD (e.g., Birmes et al., 2001; Spiegel et al., 1996). A recent 20-year review of studies using the SASRQ summarizes a good evidence base for its continued use (Lötvall et al., 2022).

Dissociation Measures

Clinicians and researchers measuring and studying dissociation have primarily used the same, nonstandardized measure (the DES-II and its predecessor, the DES) since the mid-1980s. With the inclusion of a dissociative subtype of PTSD in the *DSM-5*, the development of, and interest in, tools to effectively assess dissociation has expanded.

Dissociative Experiences Scale–II

The Dissociative Experiences Scale–II (DES-II; Carlson & Putnam, 1993), the most commonly used self-report instrument of dissociation, measures experiences such as depersonalization, derealization, amnesia, and absorption. This 28-item measure of trait dissociation is perhaps best used to screen for dissociative symptomatology. Items are rated on an 11-point scale from 0% (*never*) to 100% (*always*), with higher ratings indicating greater frequency and presumably more severe dissociation. Recommended cut scores are available when screening for dissociative disorders. However, the DES-II has received criticism for both underdiagnosing and overdiagnosing dissociative disorders (Brand et al., 2006; Ross, 2021), in terms of its response format, and the lack of accepted clinical and nonclinical norms (Dalenberg et al., 2012; Wright and Loftus, 1999). Carlson and Putnam (1993) recommended that items endorsed at the 20% level or higher be followed up on by the clinician to gather further information. Nevertheless, the DES-II and the original DES have shown good reliability and validity. Attempts to revise and improve the psychometric qualities of the scale are ongoing (e.g., Arzoumanian et al., 2023; Saggino et al., 2020).

Multidimensional Inventory of Dissociation

The Multidimensional Inventory of Dissociation (MID; Dell, 2006) consists of 218 items that yield 14 major facets of dissociation, 23 symptoms of dissociation, and 5 validity scales (Somer & Dell, 2005, p. 31). There are English (Dell, 2006) and Hebrew (Somer & Dell, 2005) versions of the MID. A study of the English version suggests that individuals with DID score higher than others on many MID scales and items (Dell, 2006). Somewhat surprisingly, given its multidimensional orientation, both the English and Hebrew versions of the MID are described as tapping a single underlying "dissociation" factor (Dell, 2006; Somer & Dell, 2005). The Hebrew version of the MID was shown to be reliable and to demonstrate convergent, discriminant, and construct validity (Somer & Dell, 2005), and the MID-80, an English short form of the MID, was found to be reliable and valid in a sample of Australian college students (Kate et al., 2021).

Dissociative Subtype of PTSD Scale

The Dissociative Subtype of PTSD Scale (DSPS; Wolf et al., 2017) measures lifetime and current dissociative symptoms using 15 items that assess the presence, frequency, and severity of the symptom. Items include symptoms from the dissociative subtype of PTSD and make up three subscales: Derealization/ Depersonalization, Loss of Awareness, and Psychogenic Amnesia. This instrument can be administered either as a self-report tool or a semistructured interview. The DSPS has strong psychometrics in samples of trauma-exposed veterans, and the Derealization/Depersonalization subscale specifically has been shown to identify the dissociative subtype of PTSD described by the *DSM-5* (Guetta et al., 2019; Wolf et al., 2017).

Somatoform Dissociation Questionnaire

The Somatoform Dissociation Questionnaire (SDQ; Nijenhuis et al., 1996) specifically evaluates symptoms involving bodily and sensory disturbances of a dissociative nature and thus differs significantly from the other dissociation measures described in this chapter. There are two versions: the SDQ-20 evaluates the severity of somatoform dissociative phenomena, whereas the SDQ-5 is a screening instrument for the presence of a dissociative disorder (Nijenhuis et al., 1997). The SDQ-20 has good reliability and convergent validity and appears to measure a coherent construct (Nijenhuis et al., 1998). The SDQ-5 demonstrated predictive validity in two studies: one demonstrating high sensitivity and specificity in discriminating dissociative disorders from other psychiatric disorders in a sample of 100 patients (.94 and .96, respectively), and one discriminating patients with DID from patients with a dissociative disorder, not otherwise specified, in a smaller (N = 31) sample (.94 and .98, respectively; Nijenhuis et al., 1997, 1998).

Trauma-Related Grief Measures

As noted in Chapter 2, our understanding of trauma-related grief has developed significantly over the past 2 decades. During this time, researchers have undertaken the measurement of traumatic grief as a construct separate from depression, general loss, or posttraumatic stress. However, one nonstandardized measure (and its revision) is especially promising, as discussed next.

Inventory of Complicated Grief–Revised

The Inventory of Complicated Grief (ICG; Prigerson et al., 1995) and its subsequent revision (the ICG-R; Prigerson & Jacobs, 2001) have demonstrated good psychometric characteristics. The ICG and the ICG-R are highly reliable, with α values in the mid to high .90s for both instruments. Furthermore, both measures have substantial content validity in the evaluation of complicated (as opposed to normal) grief responses. The 37-item ICG-R yields both a continuous total score and a dichotomous diagnosis of complicated grief.

The latter diagnosis was found in one study to have a sensitivity of .93 and a specificity of .93 in detecting interview-determined complicated grief (Barry et al., 2002). In a study of friends of people who died by suicide (Prigerson et al., 1999), those with an ICG-R determination of complicated grief had a five times greater likelihood of suicidal ideation than those without complicated grief, after controlling for depression. The ICG-R is a good example of a research measure that, were it to be normed and standardized, would be a useful clinical test.

CONCLUSION

Trauma-specific psychological tests play an important role in the complete assessment of a trauma survivor. In combination with a clinical interview, and possibly one of the broadband generic measures from Chapter 6, these tools have the potential to yield a comprehensive clinical picture. Ranging from those assessing posttraumatic and acute stress to those measuring dissociation, complex PTSD, and DSOs, these instruments help identify the quality, scope, and details of trauma-related outcomes. In doing so, they not only help us to better understand the client as a whole, but they also support treatment selection and planning, monitoring of symptom change, and overall improvements in treatment effectiveness.

Although there are numerous trauma-specific instruments now available for use, only a handful have been properly standardized and normed, and many are more appropriate for use as research measures than clinical tools, as noted earlier. An important psychometric goal for test authors and trauma researchers is to devise and further develop, validate, and standardize trauma-sensitive instruments to ensure a robust catalogue of evidence-based assessment tools.

8 TELEASSESSMENT

Although much of this book has been concerned with trauma assessment procedures conducted within an office or clinic setting, the advent of the coronavirus disease (COVID-19) pandemic in 2020 led to a significant shift in assessment (and treatment) practices for many mental health clinicians. In-person office visits became rare, and clinicians began using telephones, video devices, and, most frequently, computers to conduct psychological assessments. This shift to teleassessment was supported in part by a preexisting literature on conducting remote assessment and treatment, developed for those unable or unwilling to attend in-person sessions by virtue of disability, logistics, or anxiety or distrust about face-to-face interactions (e.g., some veterans, individuals experiencing homelessness, or people in rural environments). The pandemic vastly increased the need for teleassessment, and the potentially fatal implications of COVID-19 transmission in in-person settings heightened the need to ensure safety during the assessment process.

Although early efforts to provide teleassessment were fraught with uncertainty, psychologists and others are developing a consensus regarding the

https://doi.org/10.1037/0000452-008
Psychological Assessment of Adult Posttraumatic States: Phenomenology, Diagnosis, and Measurement, Third Edition, by E. M. Eadie and J. Briere

conduct, ethics, and technology of remote assessment. These developments and guidelines tend to focus on several areas: adherence to professional standards, technology, modalities of teleassessment, cultural and social factors, psychometric and standardization issues, choice of appropriate psychological tests, and report writing. As described in this chapter, these domains are certainly relevant when the client presents with trauma-related issues.

Importantly, this chapter only addresses in brief the foci and process of teleassessment. The reader is referred to the following resources for more detail and for professional guidelines:

- Guidelines for the Practice of Telepsychology (American Psychological Association, 2013)

- Ethical Principles of Psychologists and Code of Conduct (American Psychological Association, 2017)

- Guidance on Psychological Testing During the COVID-19 Crisis (American Psychological Association, 2020d)

- APA Guidelines for Psychological Assessment and Evaluation (American Psychological Association, 2020a)

- Ethical Guidance for the COVID-19 Era (American Psychological Association, 2020c)

- Standards for Educational and Psychological Testing (American Educational Research Association et al., 2014)

- Trauma Teletherapy for Youth in the Era of the COVID-19 Pandemic: Adapting Evidence-Based Treatment Approaches (Briere, Lanktree, & Escott, 2020)

- Teleassessment Guidance for Psychological, Psychoeducational and Neuropsychological Assessment (Educational Testing Service, n.d.)

- Best Practices for Remote Psychological Assessment via Telehealth Technologies (Luxton et al., 2014)

- Telepractice and Questionnaires or Rating Scales (Pearson, 2021)

- COVID-19 Resources: Teleassessment Resources (Society for Personality Assessment, 2023)

- COVID Task Force to Support Personality Assessment Teleassessment of Personality and Psychopathology (Society for Personality Assessment, n.d.)

ADHERENCE TO PROFESSIONAL STANDARDS

As in other professional circumstances, clinicians must adhere to high professional standards when conducting remote assessments and must follow professional, state/provincial, and federal regulations and legal requirements for teleassessment. Psychologists, in particular, must take care to follow the American Psychological Association (APA) Ethical Principles of Psychologists and Code of Conduct (American Psychological Association, 2017) and the Standards for Educational and Psychological Testing (American Educational Research Association et al., 2014).

Before formal teleassessment begins, the clinician should assess whether the client is able to tolerate remote assessment and whether it is even appropriate in the first place. As noted by the Joint Task Force for the Development of Telepsychology Guidelines for Psychologists (2013), this may include the following:

> the potential risks and benefits of providing telepsychology services for the client's/patient's particular needs, the multicultural and ethical issues that may arise, and a review of the most appropriate medium (video teleconference, text, e-mail, etc.) or best options available for the service delivery. (p. 795)

Because traumatized individuals may especially suffer from perceived lack of safety, trust issues, and, potentially, confusion regarding their entitlements in power-laden relationships, it is all the more important that the testing process be characterized by clinician trustworthiness and competence, as much transparency as possible, careful attention to confidentiality and boundaries, and fully informed consent to assessment.

Competency in Teleassessment

Because teleassessment requires the use of technology (e.g., a telephone, computer, or tablet), a platform (e.g., Zoom, Webex) compliant with the Health Insurance Portability and Accountability Act (HIPAA) of 1996 (Centers for Disease Control and Prevention, 2024), and, in many cases, a dedicated testing program, there is often a steep learning curve associated with competent remote testing. For this reason, the clinician should practice using these devices and programs until they are competent to employ them in actual clinical contexts. This practice may involve doing test runs with friends or colleagues, as well as attending courses or reading the literature on the mechanics and logistics of teleassessment. Testing clinicians also should be well-versed in, and capable of addressing, the potential pitfalls associated with teleassessment, including poor internet connections, device failures, image "freezing," distortion, pixilation, data-lagging that causes one party to inadvertently speak over the other, or sudden loss of audio and/or video signals.

Trauma clients may be more prone than others to experience such glitches as potential evidence of clinician disattunement or even abandonment or may suffer from hyperarousal-based symptoms that reduce their ability to modulate frustration or irritability when things go wrong technologically. In some cases, the trauma survivor may be hypervigilant, interpreting teleassessment interruptions or failures as evidence of maltreatment or persecution by the therapist or an intrusion by an assumed malignant entity, such as an enemy, the government, or law enforcement. For these reasons, the assessor should anticipate possible technical difficulties and be prepared to problem-solve both the logistics and the client's reactions to them.

Informed Consent

A central tenet for teleassessment, or any other clinical assessment process, is that the client be given written, understandable information about the process so that they can truly consent to psychological assessment. This information usually includes, but is not limited to, (a) what services will be performed and how they will be billed; (b) the assessment process itself, including what test instruments will be used and how testing platforms will be employed; (c) limitations of teleassessment devices and programs, including their security or lack thereof, and any other risks (e.g., hacking) associated with teleassessment; (d) how assessment results will be collected, stored, and communicated to others (including HIPAA requirements); and (e) how confidentiality will be maintained and under what conditions it can be broken.

Confidentiality

Confidentiality, one of the bedrocks of mental health practice, requires that mental health practitioners not reveal information on the client's therapy or assessment to nondesignated individuals or institutions unless there is an imminent threat to the client or someone else. In teleassessment, confidentiality also involves protections against the unauthorized communication or release of internet-transmitted data, whether misdirected, hacked, or maliciously posted audio or visual clips; violations of privacy associated with family members or others overhearing the assessment session; or leaked information from non–HIPAA-compliant communication or assessment platforms. As noted in the APA guidelines for the practice of telepsychology, clinicians who provide teleassessment must "make reasonable efforts to protect and maintain the confidentiality of the data and information relating to their clients/patients and inform them of the potentially increased risks of loss of confidentiality inherent in the use of the telecommunication technologies, if any" (American Psychological Association, 2013, p. 796).

Security of Teleassessment Platforms

With the proliferation of internet-based communication platforms, an important concern is whether confidentiality and privacy can be assured, especially whether the platform is compliant with HIPAA, which protects sensitive patient health care information from being disclosed without the patient's consent (Centers for Disease Control and Prevention, 2024). Currently, common compliant/configurable platforms include, but are not limited to, the following:

- Zoom (https://zoom.us)
- Zoom for Healthcare (https://zoom.us/healthcare)
- Doxy.me (https://doxy.me)
- Webex (https://www.webex.com)
- TheraNest (https://theranest.com)
- SimplePractice (https://simplepractice.com)
- Thera-LINK (https://www.thera-link.com)
- Microsoft Teams (https://www.microsoft.com/en-us/microsoft-teams)
- Updox (https://www.updox.com/)
- VSee (https://vsee.com)
- Google Meet (https://meet.google.com)

This list does not include FaceTime, Skype, or Facebook Messenger, which were not HIPAA compliant at the time of this writing. However, these platforms were included in an emergency notice by the U.S. Department of Health and Human Services (HHS; 2021), allowing their use during the COVID-19 pandemic. The HHS noted, however, that "providers are encouraged to notify patients that these third-party applications potentially introduce privacy risks, and providers should enable all available encryption and privacy modes when using such applications." Because this exemption expired on August 9, 2023, the reader should investigate the HIPAA acceptability of any teleassessment platform they consider using and determine what policies are currently in effect.

RAPPORT-BUILDING, ATTUNEMENT, AND SAFETY

Although there is good evidence that teleassessment can be successfully applied in various contexts (Garvin et al., 2022), client–clinician interaction via computer or telephone is a relatively constrained process that may challenge or reduce the effectiveness of the assessment relationship. For example, some clients may complain that video-based interactions do not seem "real" enough. Subtle cues and responses between the client and the evaluator may be harder to perceive, sometimes triggering the client and leading them to experience decreased interpersonal connection or hyper-vigilance to danger or disattunement (Briere, Lanktree, & Escott, 2020). As mentioned, any technical difficulties associated with video sessions can be frustrating and potentially signal danger or unpredictability. For these reasons, we suggest that, while always attending to standardization concerns, the assessor carefully communicate acceptance and support whenever problems emerge, check in with clients when it appears necessary regarding their ongoing experience during the assessment session, and reinforce the safety of the teleassessment session to the extent possible.

Specific to trauma survivors or others in potentially dangerous environments, teleassessment may inadvertently increase client danger by not establishing physical safety during the assessment process, because the client is not interviewed in the safety of the clinician's office. In general, teleassessment should be conducted in the safest, most private place in the client's environment, such as a room where the client can be alone and will not be interrupted or overheard.

We generally suggest that the client be asked about their immediate environment at the beginning of each session, including their physical address if not already known. Beyond their location, this will involve specific questions about whether the client is in any immediate danger and whether anyone else is present, answerable in a *yes* or *no* format so that any listener cannot determine the question. In some cases, the client and clinician may settle on a *danger word* that the client can insert into the teleassessment session when they are in danger or being monitored (Briere, Lanktree, & Escott, 2020).

Safety Planning

When danger cannot be ruled out, it may be helpful to explicitly plan a way for a client to escape immediate violence from an abusive caretaker or partner or from some other potentially violent or sexually exploitive person. Safety plans typically involve detailed strategies for exiting the home or environment when danger is present; access to a packed bag and, when possible, cash or a credit card; ways to contact local authorities or others who can intervene to provide safety; and names and directions to a safe place, such as a friend's home or a shelter. Much of their benefit resides in preplanning specific actions, so that when escape is necessary, the client can immediately turn to a defined strategy (Briere & Lanktree, 2012). It is also useful to inform the client ahead of time what steps the clinician will take if a safety or medical emergency becomes apparent during a teleassessment session (e.g., calling 911 and providing the client's specific address or location if it is safe to do so).

CULTURAL AND SOCIAL FACTORS

As the APA teleassessment guidelines suggest, it is important for clinicians to make "reasonable efforts to understand the manner in which cultural, linguistic, socioeconomic, and other individual characteristics (e.g., medical status, psychiatric stability, physical/cognitive disability, personal preferences)" (American Psychological Association, 2020d, p. 794) may potentially affect the client's full access to competent psychological testing. As noted by Luxton and colleagues (2014), teleassessment may miss or discourage disclosure regarding symptomatology, dysfunction, or distress among individuals living in cultures or subcultures that emphasize interpersonal connectedness or rely heavily on nonverbal reactions, as well as among those who tend to be more technologically naïve. In addition, marginalized people and those experiencing poverty may have less access to computers or other teleassessment devices, and those living in cultures that do not share Western models of psychological illness may employ idioms of distress (see Chapter 3, this volume) that are not well tapped by Eurocentric tests and measures, whether through teleassessment or otherwise. In such cases, the clinician should consider sociocultural issues when deciding the relevance of teleassessment to any specific client, and, when appropriate, employ measures more relevant to the experiences of marginalized clients or utilize a brief questionnaire or interview (e.g., the Harvard Trauma Questionnaire; Mollica et al., 1996) that takes cultural variation into account. When these options are also unsuccessful or contraindicated, the assessor may choose to utilize a communication platform to engage in a more culturally relevant, albeit informal, interview about the client's mental health concerns.

PSYCHOMETRIC AND STANDARDIZATION ISSUES

Administration of tests and standardized interviews in a teleassessment environment can differ in important ways from those in which they were initially normed and standardized. For example, a test inventory may have been standardized on respondents who read test items and physically record their responses on an answer sheet. In a teleassessment context, however, test administration may be digital, and the client may complete the test on their personal computer—reading items and entering their own responses, which are then automatically sent back to the clinician by the testing platform. Or, in some cases, the assessment may vary more significantly from the standardization set, with the clinician reading test items aloud, the client responding verbally, and the clinician then recording the responses. These variations may alter the meaning of client's responses and may make it more difficult to compare the extremity of their results to existing normative data.

Nonstandardized assessment during teleassessment also may easily alter the psychometrics of psychological tests, because changes to the original assessment process may reduce the reliability and/or validity of measures assessed in more controlled environments. For example, a scale that is internally consistent and correlated with relevant variables in the standardization sample may be less psychometrically acceptable when the items are read to the client, paraphrased in an interview, provided in nonstandardized contexts, or administered to individuals whose demographic and cultural characteristics are not equivalent to those in the standardization sample.

Standardization issues in teleassessment can be at least partially addressed in several ways, including using tests developed for teleassessment, administering written tests verbally, and using interview-based assessments. Some specific recommendations are outlined next.

1. Administer Tests That Have Been Adapted for Telehealth Settings

Some psychological test companies have developed online assessment packages wherein test items are presented to the client online, the client clicks or otherwise indicates their answer on an online answer sheet, and then these responses are transmitted back to the clinician or the assessment company. In such cases, the standardization requirements of the test are essentially met, because the process involves clicks or typed responses to textual items and the clinician is not directly involved. Although this solution can be a good one, not all relevant psychological tests have been adapted for online administration.

2. Verbally Administer Existing Written Tests Online

Although administration of existing written tests verbally through an online platform is not uncommon in teletherapy contexts, it can be problematic to the extent that it is unclear whether a given client symptom endorsement reflects solely their response to a given test item or also includes reactivity to verbally sharing responses with the clinician. For example, items that ask about potentially embarrassing or socially inappropriate behaviors might be endorsed at lower levels when they are reported verbally to the therapist, as opposed to in a noninteractive, written context.

3. Use Assessment Instruments That Are Interview Based or Do Not Rely on Standardized Normative Comparisons

In the case of interviews, the standardization requirements are typically met: The initial measure was based on verbally asking clients questions, and the clinician does the same, albeit through the internet as opposed to an office session. The clinician may also administer tests that have not been classically standardized and do not yield statistically based conclusions. In such instances, the clinician usually reads test items to the client during the teleassessment session and records their verbal responses or uses the screen-sharing option in video platforms such as Zoom. In this latter case, clients can read the items on their screens (as opposed to having the clinician read to them), and then indicate their responses to the therapist. Such tests are often used on a descriptive basis and for screening purposes, and they typically are not as clinically interpretable as standardized tests.

Whatever the adaptation, the mental health professional must describe and disclose any modifications or alterations made to the standardization procedures associated with a given psychological measure and consider the impact of these differences on the relevance, reliability, validity, and interpretability of the client's test scores. The reader is referred to the APA telepsychology guidelines, which encourage assessors to account for "the potential difference between the results obtained when a particular psychological test is conducted via telepsychology and when it is administered in-person" and to specify in any subsequent written report "that a particular test or assessment procedure has been administered via telepsychology, and describe any accommodations or modifications that have been made" (American Psychological Association, 2024).

REPORT WRITING

As described by the Educational Testing Service (n.d.), psychological reports based on teleassessment should include the following:

- the location(s) where the assessment was conducted (i.e., the location of the evaluator, as well as the test taker);

- the communication and assessment platforms used and whether they were HIPAA compliant;

- if the assessment was a hybrid of in-person and teleassessment, which aspects of the assessment were conducted in person, and which were conducted via teleassessment; and

- whether there were any technology disruptions or other situational factors that may have impacted the psychometric quality or interpretability of the assessment process.

Any alterations and modifications to standard procedures should be identified in the assessment report and feedback session as discussed earlier, as well as any implications for test interpretation. In this regard, examiners should ensure the "conditions of administration indicated in the test manual are preserved when adapted for use with such technologies" (Joint Task Force for the Development of Telepsychology Guidelines for Psychologists, 2013, p. 798).

A typical report, adapted from the Pearson (2021) guidelines on reporting teleassessment results, might state something like this:

> The following tests were administered via remote teleassessment: [*list of measures*], using the [*name of communication platform (e.g., Zoom)*] platform. Measures were administered from the clinician's office and completed in the client's home. [*If true*] The remote testing environment appeared free of distractions, adequate rapport was established with the examinee via video/audio, and the examinee appeared appropriately engaged in the task throughout the session. [*If true*] No significant technological problems or distractions were noted during administration. Modifications to the standardization procedure included: [*list if any*].

CONCLUSION

Although the heavy reliance on teleassessment services that occurred during the initial phase of the COVID-19 pandemic has now abated and many services have returned to in-person, in-clinic settings, it is likely that the expansion and formalization of teleassessment procedures and practices described in this chapter will remain. These technological adaptations will no doubt continue to have widespread benefit, especially for rural and remote clients as well as those who are limited in mobility or otherwise reluctant to attend in-person services.

9

CONCLUSION

The pervasiveness of trauma, in its many forms, is a difficult reality to grasp. Interpersonal violence, war, mass shootings, accidents, disasters, hate crimes, and pandemic viral disease are regular aspects of modern human existence. Since the publication of the *Diagnostic and Statistical Manual of Mental Disorders, Third Edition* (*DSM-III*; American Psychiatric Association, 1980), many thousands of articles, chapters, and books have been written on the epidemiology, etiology, assessment, and treatment of posttraumatic symptoms, problems, and disorders. At the same time, a new branch of mental health specialty has emerged, with its primary focus being the assessment, diagnosis, and treatment of trauma-related difficulties. Researchers and clinicians have discovered a collection of psychological outcomes that are intrinsically related to traumatic events yet have been largely overlooked in the past. These include acute stress disorder, posttraumatic stress disorder, brief psychotic disorder, the adjustment disorders, dissociative disorders, somatization disorders, personality disorders, and difficulties in identity, relatedness, and self-regulation that arise from early traumatic events. With each additional

https://doi.org/10.1037/0000452-009
Psychological Assessment of Adult Posttraumatic States: *Phenomenology, Diagnosis, and Measurement, Third Edition,* by E. M. Eadie and J. Briere

iteration of the *DSM* diagnostic system (i.e., the progression from *DSM-I* to *DSM-5-TR*; American Psychiatric Association, 1952, 2022), these outcomes have become more clearly defined, although there may have been some errors along the way. So, too, has our understanding grown of the complex interaction between genetics, social status, life history, single and cumulative stressors, and the environment in the genesis of posttraumatic disturbance.

We have also come to realize that traumatic events can involve not only fear of death and severe disability, as stressed in the various *DSM* editions, but also major adverse phenomena that do not meet *DSM-5-TR* criteria. These events include early acts of omission, such as severe childhood neglect and parental disattunement, as well as exposure to racism, sexism, anti-LGBTQ+ behaviors, and forms of xenophobia such as antisemitism, Islamophobia, and anti-immigrant violence. This book has considered one small piece of this growing knowledge base: the accurate and reliable assessment of posttraumatic outcomes.

Throughout this volume, we have highlighted many of the strengths, limitations, and gaps in current assessment practice and existing trauma assessment tools. Traditional psychological tests have tended to misinterpret posttraumatic symptoms, often identifying them as psychosis, personality disorder, and other less relevant psychological conditions or dismissing them as feigned or exaggerated states. The net effect has been to provide potentially erroneous information to clinicians, sometimes leading to inadequate treatment and prolonged suffering. Moreover, many trauma-specific tests and inventories have failed to capture the full range of posttraumatic symptoms and experiences, potentially leaving the novice clinician with the impression that classic posttraumatic stress is the only area to look out for and measure.

Advancing the field of trauma assessment requires a concerted effort to develop and validate tools that not only meet rigorous research standards but also translate effectively into clinical practice. This includes integrating a broader range of relational, dissociative, somatic, and self-regulation issues into trauma assessment tools. Furthermore, although many of the scales reviewed in Chapter 7 have acceptable psychometrics, they lack the normative data required to ensure effective interpretation.

Fortunately, we are continuously improving our understanding of the phenomenology of posttraumatic disturbance and are increasingly able to provide assessment approaches that accurately tap the internal experience of the trauma survivor. Clinicians have adapted traditional psychological tests to better assess posttraumatic outcomes, often by developing new scoring systems and interpretation approaches, and by creating more trauma-sensitive scales within these measures. Even more important is the development of a host of new standardized psychological tests and struc-tured interviews that directly assess trauma and its impacts. As a result, trauma survivors in both mental health and emergency-outreach populations are increasingly likely to be understood clinically—an outcome that can only lead to improved intervention and a greater likelihood of recovery.

BROADBAND TRAUMA/ADVERSITY REVIEW (BTAR)

1. <u>Before you were age 18</u>, did a parent or another adult who was in charge of you ever hurt or punish you in a way that left a bruise, cut, scratches, or broken bones or teeth or made you bleed?

   Yes __ No __

   If yes:

   Did you ever think you might be injured or killed?

   Yes __ No __

2. <u>Before you were age 18</u>, were you ever physically attacked, assaulted, stabbed, shot at, or otherwise physically hurt by someone who wasn't a parent or another adult in charge of you?

   Yes __ No __

   If yes:

   Did this ever happen with a boyfriend, girlfriend, sex partner, or spouse?

   Yes __ No __

   Did you ever think you might be injured or killed?

   Yes __ No __

3. <u>Before you were age 18</u>, was something sexual ever done to you against your will or when you couldn't defend yourself (for example, when you were asleep or intoxicated)?

   Yes __ No __

If yes:

Was this ever done by a parent or someone else in charge of you?

Yes __ No __

Did this ever happen on a date, or with a sexual/romantic partner or spouse?

Yes __ No __

Did you ever think you might be injured or killed?

Yes __ No __

4. Before you were age 18, how often did at least one of your parents or another adult who were in charge of you yell at you, criticize you, say mean things to you, or put you down?

Never		Sometimes		Very often
1	2	3	4	5

5. Before you were age 18, how often did at least one of your parents or another adult who was in charge of you act "spaced out" around you, didn't pay attention to you, or didn't notice when you were upset or needed something?

Never		Sometimes		Very often
1	2	3	4	5

6. Before you were age 18, were you ever homeless (for example, living on the streets, in a car, in a park, at a bus or train station, or in a shelter)?

Yes __ No __

If yes:

Did you ever think you might be injured or killed?

Yes __ No __

7. Before you were age 18, did your parents or some else in charge of you ever neglect you by not providing enough food, clean clothes, medical or dental treatment, or a safe place to stay, even though they probably could have taken better care of you?

Yes __ No __

8. <u>Before you were age 18</u>, was your family ever very poor, on welfare, or getting public assistance?

   Yes __ No __

9. <u>Before you were age 18</u>, did you ever get so sick that you thought you might die?

   Yes __ No __

10. <u>Before you were age 18</u>, were you ever involved in a serious automobile accident?

    Yes __ No __

    If yes:

    Did you ever think you might be injured or killed?

    Yes __ No __

11. <u>Before you were age 18</u>, were you ever involved in a serious fire, major earthquake, flood, or other disaster?

    Yes __ No __

    If yes:

    Did you ever think you might be injured or killed?

    Yes __ No __

12. <u>Before you were age 18</u>, did you ever see someone else get killed, beaten, or badly hurt?

    Yes __ No __

    If yes:

    Did you ever see this ever happen to a friend, relative, or loved one?

    Yes __ No __

13. <u>Before you were age 18</u>, were you ever hit, beaten, assaulted, or shot by the police, border patrol, or other law enforcement officials during or after an arrest or at some other time?

    Yes __ No __

If yes:

Did you ever think you might be injured or killed?

Yes __ No __

14. <u>Before you were age 18</u>, were you discriminated against or mistreated by people because of your sex, race or ethnicity, gender identity, sexual orientation, or religion?

Never		Sometimes		Very often
1	2	3	4	5

If yes:

Did you ever think you might be injured or killed?

Yes __ No __

15. <u>Before you were age 18</u>, did anyone ever repeatedly follow you around or stalk you to the extent that you felt intimidated or threatened?

Yes __ No __

If yes:

Did you ever think you might be injured or killed?

Yes __ No __

16. <u>Before you were age 18</u>, did a parent or some other adult in charge of you regularly drink too much or take serious drugs?

Yes __ No __

17. <u>Before you were age 18</u>, did a parent or some other adult in charge of you ever go to prison or jail?

Yes __ No __

18. <u>Before you were age 18</u>, were you ever in foster care or a foster home?

Yes __ No __

19. <u>Before you were age 18</u>, did anything else ever happen to you that was very upsetting or made you afraid you would be badly hurt or killed?

Yes __ No __

If yes:

Please describe what happened:

20. <u>Since you were age 18 or older,</u> have you ever been physically attacked, assaulted, stabbed, shot at, or otherwise physically hurt by someone?

    Yes __ No __

    If yes:

    Did this ever happen with a boyfriend, girlfriend, sex partner, or spouse?

    Yes __ No __

    Did you ever think you might be injured or killed?

    Yes __ No __

21. <u>Since you were age 18 or older,</u> has something sexual ever been done to you against your will or when you couldn't defend yourself (for example, when you were asleep or intoxicated)?

    Yes __ No __

    If yes:

    Did this ever happen with a boyfriend, girlfriend, sex partner, or spouse?

    Yes __ No __

    Did you ever think you might be injured or killed?

    Yes __ No __

22. <u>Since you were age 18 or older,</u> have you ever been in a war?

    Yes __ No __

    If yes:

    Were you ever injured?

    Yes __ No __

    Did you ever think you might be injured or killed?

    Yes __ No __

23. <u>Since you were age 18 or older,</u> have you ever been involved in a serious automobile accident?

    Yes __ No __

    If yes:

    Did you ever think you might be injured or killed?

24. <u>Since you were age 18 or older,</u> have you ever been involved in a serious fire, major earthquake, flood, or other disaster?

    Yes __ No __

    If yes:

    Did you ever think you might be injured or killed?

    Yes __ No __

25. <u>Since you were age 18 or older,</u> have you ever been homeless (for example, living on the streets, in a car, in a park, at a bus or train station, or in a shelter)?

    Yes __ No __

    If yes:

    Did you ever think you might be injured or killed?

    Yes __ No __

26. <u>Since you were age 18 or older,</u> in the United States or another country, have you ever been tortured by the government or by people against the government?

    Yes __ No __

    If yes:

    Did you ever think you might be injured or killed?

    Yes __ No __

27. <u>Since you were age 18 or older,</u> have you ever been hit, beaten, assaulted, or shot by the police, border patrol, or other law enforcement officials during or after an arrest or at some other time?

    Yes __ No __

If yes:

Did you ever think you might be injured or killed?

Yes __ No __

28. <u>Since you were age 18 or older</u>, have you ever seen someone else killed, beaten, or badly hurt?

Yes __ No __

If yes:

Did you ever see this happen to a friend, relative, or loved one?

Yes __ No __

29. <u>Since you were age 18 or older</u>, has anyone ever followed you around or stalked you to the extent that you felt intimidated or threatened?

Yes __ No __

If yes:

Did you ever think you might be injured or killed?

Yes __ No __

30. <u>Since you were age 18 or older</u>, have you been discriminated against or mistreated because of your sex, race or ethnicity, gender identity, sexual orientation, or religion?

Never		Sometimes		Very often
1	2	3	4	5

If yes:

Did you ever think you might be injured or killed?

Yes __ No __

31. <u>Since you were age 18 or older</u>, have you ever gotten so sick that you thought you might die?

Yes __ No __

32. <u>Since you were age 18 or older</u>, have you ever had to go to prison or jail?

Yes __ No __

If yes:

For how long?

Less than a month____   Between a month and a year____
More than a year but   5 years or longer____
  less than 5 years____

33. <u>Since you were age 18 or older,</u> has anything else ever happened to you that was very upsetting or made you afraid you would be badly hurt or killed?

Yes __ No __

If yes:

Please describe what happened:

Appendix B

SOCIAL DISCRIMINATION AND MALTREATMENT SCALE–SHORT FORM

Please rate how often the following things have happened in your life, because of how people responded to your *sex*, *race*, or *sexual orientation or gender identity*. If it has never happened to you, circle "1." If it has happened very often, circle "5."

1. I have been discriminated against Never   Very often
  a. Because of my sex   1   2   3   4   5
  b. Because of my race   1   2   3   4   5
  c. Because of my sexual orientation   1   2   3   4   5
    or gender identity

2. I have been unsafe   Never   Very often
  a. Because of my sex   1   2   3   4   5
  b. Because of my race   1   2   3   4   5
  c. Because of my sexual orientation   1   2   3   4   5
    or gender identity

3. People made cruel or demeaning jokes about me   Never   Very often
  a. Because of my sex   1   2   3   4   5
  b. Because of my race   1   2   3   4   5
  c. Because of my sexual orientation   1   2   3   4   5
    or gender identity

4. I have felt powerless	**Never**			**Very often**	
a. Because of my sex	1	2	3	4	5
b. Because of my race	1	2	3	4	5
c. Because of my sexual orientation or gender identity	1	2	3	4	5

5. I have felt like people were judging me	**Never**			**Very often**	
a. Because of my sex	1	2	3	4	5
b. Because of my race	1	2	3	4	5
c. Because of my sexual orientation or gender identity	1	2	3	4	5

6. I have been disrespected	**Never**			**Very often**	
a. Because of my sex	1	2	3	4	5
b. Because of my race	1	2	3	4	5
c. Because of my sexual orientation or gender identity	1	2	3	4	5

References

Acierno, R., Hernandez, M. A., Amstadter, A. B., Resnick, H. S., Steve, K., Muzzy, W., & Kilpatrick, D. G. (2010). Prevalence and correlates of emotional, physical, sexual, and financial abuse and potential neglect in the United States: The National Elder Mistreatment Study. *American Journal of Public Health, 100*(2), 292–297. https://doi.org/10.2105/AJPH.2009.163089

Adams, R. S., Nikitin, R. V., Wooten, N. R., Williams, T. V., & Larson, M. J. (2016). The association of combat exposure with postdeployment behavioral health problems among U.S. Army enlisted women returning from Afghanistan or Iraq. *Journal of Traumatic Stress, 29*(4), 356–364. https://doi.org/10.1002/jts.22121

Akagi, H., & House, A. (2002). The clinical epidemiology of hysteria: Vanishingly rare, or just vanishing? *Psychological Medicine, 32*(2), 191–194. https://doi.org/10.1017/S0033291701004962

Ales, F., & Erdodi, L. (2022). Detecting negative response bias within the Trauma Symptom Inventory–2 (TSI-2): A review of the literature. *Psychological Injury and Law, 15*(1), 56–63. https://doi.org/10.1007/s12207-021-09427-9

Alford, C. F. (2016). *Trauma, culture, and PTSD*. Palgrave Macmillan US. https://doi.org/10.1057/978-1-137-57600-2

Allen, B. (2011). Childhood psychological abuse and adult aggression: The mediating role of self-capacities. *Journal of Interpersonal Violence, 26*(10), 2093–2110. https://doi.org/10.1177/0886260510383035

Allen, J. G., Coyne, L., & Console, D. A. (1997). Dissociative detachment relates to psychotic symptoms and personality decompensation. *Comprehensive Psychiatry, 38*(6), 327–334. https://doi.org/10.1016/S0010-440X(97)90928-7

Allen, J. G., Coyne, L., & Huntoon, J. (1998). Complex posttraumatic stress disorder in women from a psychometric perspective. *Journal of Personality Assessment, 70*(2), 277–298. https://doi.org/10.1207/s15327752jpa7002_7

Allen, J. G., Huntoon, J., & Evans, R. B. (1999). Complexities in complex posttraumatic stress disorder in inpatient women: Evidence from cluster analysis of MCMI-III Personality Disorder Scales. *Journal of Personality Assessment*, *73*(3), 449–471. https://doi.org/10.1207/S15327752JPA7303_10

Allwood, M., Ghafoori, B., Salgado, C., Slobodin, O., Kreither, J., Waelde, L. C., Larrondo, P., & Ramos, N. (2022). Identity-based hate and violence as trauma: Current research, clinical implications, and advocacy in a globally connected world. *Journal of Traumatic Stress*, *35*(2), 349–361. https://doi.org/10.1002/jts.22748

Alpher, V. S. (1991). Assessment of ego functioning in multiple personality disorder. *Journal of Personality Assessment*, *56*, 373–387.

Álvarez, M.-J., Roura, P., Osés, A., Foguet, Q., Solà, J., & Arrufat, F.-X. (2011). Prevalence and clinical impact of childhood trauma in patients with severe mental disorders. *Journal of Nervous and Mental Disease*, *199*(3), 156–161. https://doi.org/10.1097/NMD.0b013e31820c751c

Amar, M. B. (2006). Cannabinoids in medicine: A review of their therapeutic potential. *Journal of Ethnopharmacology*, *105*(1–2), 1–25. https://doi.org/10.1016/j.jep.2006.02.001

Ambrose, T., Giarratano, K. J., McCue, M. L., Brand, B. L., & Dalenberg, C. J. (2025). Utility of the Minnesota Multiphasic Personality Inventory-2 in differentiating genuine from feigned dissociative identity disorder. *Psychological Trauma: Theory, Research, Practice, and Policy*, *17*(2), 307–315. https://doi.org/10.1037/tra0001611

American Academy of Clinical Neuropsychology. (2021). *Position statement on use of race as a factor in neuropsychological test norming and performance prediction.* https://theaacn.org/wp-content/uploads/2021/11/AACN-Position-Statement-on-Race-Norms.pdf

American Burn Association. (2024). *Burn Injury Summary Report (BISR).* https://ameriburn.org/quality-care/burn-care-quality-platform-bcqp-registry/bcqp-bisr/

American Educational Research Association, American Psychological Association, & National Council on Measurement in Education. (Eds.). (2014). *Standards for educational and psychological testing.* American Educational Research Association.

American Psychiatric Association. (1952). *Diagnostic and statistical manual of mental disorders.*

American Psychiatric Association. (1968). *Diagnostic and statistical manual of mental disorders* (2nd ed.).

American Psychiatric Association. (1980). *Diagnostic and statistical manual of mental disorders* (3rd ed.).

American Psychiatric Association. (1987). *Diagnostic and statistical manual of mental disorders* (3rd ed., rev).

American Psychiatric Association. (1994). *Diagnostic and statistical manual of mental disorders* (4th ed.).

American Psychiatric Association. (2000). *Diagnostic and statistical manual of mental disorders* (4th ed., text rev.).

American Psychiatric Association. (2013). *Diagnostic and statistical manual of mental disorders* (5th ed.).

American Psychiatric Association. (2017). *Mental health disparities: Women's mental health.* https://www.psychiatry.org/getmedia/aa325a61-5b60-4c71-80f1-dc80cf83c383/Mental-Health-Facts-for-Women.pdf

American Psychiatric Association. (2020). *Moral injury during the COVID-19 pandemic.* https://www.psychiatry.org/File%20Library/Psychiatrists/APA-Guidance-COVID-19-Moral-Injury.pdf

American Psychiatric Association. (2022). *Diagnostic and statistical manual of mental disorders* (5th ed., text rev.).

American Psychiatric Association. (2024). *What is somatic symptom disorder?* https://www.psychiatry.org/patients-families/somatic-symptom-disorder/what-is-somatic-symptom-disorder

American Psychological Association. (n.d.). *Psychological and neuropsychological assessment with transgender and gender nonbinary adults.* https://www.apa.org/pi/lgbt/resources/transgender-gender-nonbinary

American Psychological Association. (2013). *Guidelines for the practice of telepsychology.* https://www.apa.org/pubs/journals/features/amp-a0035001.pdf

American Psychological Association. (2017). *Ethical principles of psychologists and code of conduct* (2002, Amended June 1, 2010, and January 1, 2017). https://www.apa.org/ethics/code/index.aspx

American Psychological Association. (2019). *Race and ethnicity guidelines in psychology: Promoting responsiveness and equity.* https://www.apa.org/about/policy/race-and-ethnicity-in-psychology.pdf

American Psychological Association. (2020a). *APA guidelines for psychological assessment and evaluation.* https://www.apa.org/about/policy/guidelines-psychological-assessment-evaluation.pdf

American Psychological Association. (2020b). *Elder abuse: How to spot warning signs, get help, and report mistreatment.* https://www.apa.org/topics/aging-older-adults/elder-abuse

American Psychological Association. (2020c). *Ethical guidance for the COVID-19 era.* https://www.apa.org/ethics/covid-19-guidance

American Psychological Association. (2020d). *Guidance on psychological tele-assessment during the COVID-19 crisis.* https://www.apaservices.org/practice/reimbursement/health-codes/testing/tele-assessment-covid-19

American Psychological Association. (2024). *Telehealth and telepsychology.* https://www.apa.org/practice/telehealth-telepsychology

American Psychological Association, APA Task Force on Psychological Practice With Sexual Minority Persons. (2021). *Guidelines for psychological practice with sexual minority persons.* https://www.apa.org/about/policy/psychological-sexual-minority-persons.pdf

Amnesty International. (2015, June 22). *Torture around the world: What you need to know.* https://www.amnesty.org/en/latest/news/2015/06/torture-around-the-world/

Anders, S. L., Frazier, P. A., & Frankfurt, S. B. (2011). Variations in Criterion A and PTSD rates in a community sample of women. *Journal of Anxiety Disorders*, *25*(2), 176–184. https://doi.org/10.1016/j.janxdis.2010.08.018

Anderson, M. C., Ochsner, K. N., Kuhl, B., Cooper, J., Robertson, E., Gabrieli, S. W., Glover, G. H., & Gabrieli, J. D. (2004). Neural systems underlying the suppression of unwanted memories. *Science*, *303*(5655), 232–235. https://doi.org/10.1126/science.1089504

Andrews, B., Brewin, C. R., Rose, S., & Kirk, M. (2000). Predicting PTSD symptoms in victims of violent crime: The role of shame, anger, and childhood abuse. *Journal of Abnormal Psychology*, *109*(1), 69–73. https://doi.org/10.1037/0021-843X.109.1.69

Aparcero, M., Picard, E. H., Nijdam-Jones, A., & Rosenfeld, B. (2023). Comparing the ability of MMPI-2 and MMPI-2-RF validity scales to detect feigning: A meta-analysis. *Assessment*, *30*(3), 744–760. https://doi.org/10.1177/10731911211067535

Arata, C. M., Saunders, B. E., & Kilpatrick, D. G. (1991). Concurrent validity of a crime-related post-traumatic stress disorder scale for women within the Symptom Checklist-90—Revised. *Violence and Victims*, *6*(3), 191–199. https://doi.org/10.1891/0886-6708.6.3.191

Arbisi, P. A. (2006). Use of the MMPI-2 in personal injury and disability evaluations. In J. N. Butcher (Ed.), *MMPI-2: A practitioner's guide* (pp. 407–441). American Psychological Association. https://doi.org/10.1037/11287-015

Armenta, R. F., Walter, K. H., Geronimo-Hara, T. R., Porter, B., Stander, V. A., LeardMann, C. A., & the Millennium Cohort Study Team. (2019). Longitudinal trajectories of comorbid PTSD and depression symptoms among U.S. service members and veterans. *BMC Psychiatry*, *19*(1), 396. https://doi.org/10.1186/s12888-019-2375-1

Armstrong, J., & Kaser-Boyd, N. (2004). Projective assessment of psychological trauma. In M. J. Hilsenroth & D. L. Segal (Eds.), *Comprehensive handbook of psychological assessment: Vol. 2. Personality assessment* (pp. 500–512). John Wiley & Sons.

Armstrong, J. G., & Loewenstein, R. J. (1990). Characteristics of patients with multiple personality and dissociative disorders on psychological testing. *Journal of Nervous and Mental Disease*, *178*, 448–454.

Arzoumanian, M. A., Verbeck, E. G., Estrellado, J. E., Thompson, K. J., Dahlin, K., Hennrich, E. J., Stevens, J. M., Dalenberg, C. J., & Trauma Research Institute. (2023). Psychometrics of three dissociation scales: Reliability and validity data on the DESR, DES-II, and DESC. *Journal of Trauma & Dissociation*, *24*(2), 214–228. https://doi.org/10.1080/15299732.2022.2119633

Avina, C., & O'Donohue, W. (2002). Sexual harassment and PTSD: Is sexual harassment diagnosable trauma? *Journal of Traumatic Stress*, *15*(1), 69–75. https://doi.org/10.1023/A:1014387429057

Aviram, R. B., Brodsky, B. S., & Stanley, B. (2006). Borderline personality disorder, stigma, and treatment implications. *Harvard Review of Psychiatry, 14*(5), 249–256. https://doi.org/10.1080/10673220600975121

Ayazi, T., Lien, L., Eide, A., Swartz, L., & Hauff, E. (2014). Association between exposure to traumatic events and anxiety disorders in a post-conflict setting: A cross-sectional community study in South Sudan. *BMC Psychiatry, 14*(1), 6. https://doi.org/10.1186/1471-244X-14-6

Bachem, R., Levin, Y., Zerach, G., Cloitre, M., & Solomon, Z. (2021). The interpersonal implications of PTSD and complex PTSD: The role of disturbances in self-organization. *Journal of Affective Disorders, 290,* 149–156. https://doi.org/10.1016/j.jad.2021.04.075

Bailey, T. D., Boyer, S. M., & Brand, B. L. (2019). Dissociative disorders. In D. L. Segal (Ed.), *Diagnostic interviewing* (pp. 401–424). Springer. https://doi.org/10.1007/978-1-4939-9127-3_16

Balsam, K. F., Beadnell, B., & Molina, Y. (2013). The Daily Heterosexist Experiences Questionnaire: Measuring minority stress among lesbian, gay, bisexual, and transgender adults. *Measurement & Evaluation in Counseling & Development, 46*(1), 3–25. https://doi.org/10.1177/0748175612449743

Barlow, D. H., Farchione, T. J., Bullis, J. R., Gallagher, M. W., Murray-Latin, H., Sauer-Zavala, S., Bentley, K. H., Thompson-Hollands, J., Conklin, L. R., Boswell, J. F., Ametaj, A., Carl, J. R., Boettcher, H. T., & Cassiello-Robbins, C. (2017). The unified protocol for transdiagnostic treatment of emotional disorders compared with diagnosis-specific protocols for anxiety disorders: A randomized clinical trial. *JAMA Psychiatry, 74*(9), 875–884. https://doi.org/10.1001/jamapsychiatry.2017.2164

Barnes, A., & Ephross, P. H. (1994). The impact of hate violence on victims: Emotional and behavioral responses to attacks. *Social Work, 39*(3), 247–251.

Barry, L. C., Kasl, S. V., & Prigerson, H. G. (2002). Psychiatric disorders among bereaved persons: The role of perceived circumstances of death and preparedness for death. *The American Journal of Geriatric Psychiatry, 10*(4), 447–457. https://doi.org/10.1097/00019442-200207000-00011

Bassuk, E., Perloff, J., & Dawson, R. (2001). Multiply homeless families: The insidious impact of violence. *Housing Policy Debates, 12,* 299–320.

Bebbington, P., Jonas, S., Kuipers, E., King, M., Cooper, C., Brugha, T., Meltzer, H., McManus, S., & Jenkins, R. (2011). Childhood sexual abuse and psychosis: Data from a cross-sectional national psychiatric survey in England. *The British Journal of Psychiatry, 199*(1), 29–37. https://doi.org/10.1192/bjp.bp.110.083642

Beck, A. T., & Steer, R. A. (1993). *Beck Anxiety Inventory manual.* Psychological Corporation.

Beckham, J. C., Moore, S. D., Feldman, M. E., Hertzberg, M. A., Kirby, A. C., & Fairbank, J. A. (1998). Health status, somatization, and severity of posttraumatic stress disorder in Vietnam combat veterans with posttraumatic stress disorder. *The American Journal of Psychiatry, 155*(11), 1565–1569. https://doi.org/10.1176/ajp.155.11.1565

Bell, K. J. (2009). A feminist's argument on how sex work can benefit women. *Inquiries, 209*, 1–2.

Bell, M. D. (1995). *Bell Object Relations and Reality Testing Inventory*. Western Psychological Services.

Bellet, B. W., McDevitt-Murphy, M. E., Thomas, D. H., & Luciano, M. T. (2018). The utility of the Personality Assessment Inventory in the assessment of posttraumatic stress disorder in OEF/OIF/OND veterans. *Assessment, 25*(8), 1074–1083. https://doi.org/10.1177/1073191116681627

Ben-Porath, Y. S., & Tellegen, A. (2008). *Minnesota Multiphasic Personality Inventory-2 Restructured Form: Manual for administration, scoring, and interpretation*. University of Minnesota Press.

Ben-Porath, Y. S., & Tellegen, A. (2020). *Minnesota Multiphasic Personality Inventory-3 (MMPI-3): Manual for administration, scoring, and interpretation*. University of Minnesota Press.

Benjet, C., Bromet, E., Karam, E. G., Kessler, R. C., McLaughlin, K. A., Ruscio, A. M., Shahly, V., Stein, D. J., Petukhova, M., Hill, E., Alonso, J., Atwoli, L., Bunting, B., Bruffaerts, R., Caldas-de-Almeida, J. M., de Girolamo, G., Florescu, S., Gureje, O., Huang, Y., . . . Koenen, K. C. (2016). The epidemiology of traumatic event exposure worldwide: Results from the World Mental Health Survey Consortium. *Psychological Medicine, 46*(2), 327–343. https://doi.org/10.1017/S0033291715001981

Bentall, R. P., Wickham, S., Shevlin, M., & Varese, F. (2012). Do specific early-life adversities lead to specific symptoms of psychosis? A study from the 2007 Adult Psychiatric Morbidity Survey. *Schizophrenia Bulletin, 38*(4), 734–740. https://doi.org/10.1093/schbul/sbs049

Berger, A. M., Knutson, J. F., Mehm, J. G., & Perkins, K. A. (1988). The self-report of punitive childhood experiences of young adults and adolescents. *Child Abuse & Neglect, 12*(2), 251–262. https://doi.org/10.1016/0145-2134(88)90033-6

Berger, W., Coutinho, E. S. F., Figueira, I., Marques-Portella, C., Luz, M. P., Neylan, T. C., Marmar, C. R., & Mendlowicz, M. V. (2012). Rescuers at risk: A systematic review and meta-regression analysis of the worldwide current prevalence and correlates of PTSD in rescue workers. *Social Psychiatry and Psychiatric Epidemiology, 47*(6), 1001–1011. https://doi.org/10.1007/s00127-011-0408-2

Berliner, L., & Briere, J. (1998). Trauma, memory, and clinical practice. In L. Williams (Ed.), *Trauma and memory* (pp. 3–18). Sage.

Berman, H., Girón, E. R., & Marroquín, A. P. (2006). A narrative study of refugee women who have experienced violence in the context of war. *Canadian Journal of Nursing Research, 38*(4), 32–53.

Bernstein, D. P., Ahluvalia, T., Pogge, D., & Handelsman, L. (1997). Validity of the Childhood Trauma Questionnaire in an adolescent psychiatric population.

Journal of the American Academy of Child and Adolescent Psychiatry, 36(3), 340–348. https://doi.org/10.1097/00004583-199703000-00012

Bernstein, D. P., Fink, L., Handelsman, L., Foote, J., Lovejoy, M., Wenzel, K., Sapareto, E., & Ruggiero, J. (1994). Initial reliability and validity of a new retrospective measure of child abuse and neglect. *The American Journal of Psychiatry, 151*(8), 1132–1136. https://doi.org/10.1176/ajp.151.8.1132

Bernstein, D. P., Stein, J. A., Newcomb, M. D., Walker, E., Pogge, D., Ahluvalia, T., Stokes, J., Handelsman, L., Medrano, M., Desmond, D., & Zule, W. (2003). Development and validation of a brief screening version of the Childhood Trauma Questionnaire. *Child Abuse & Neglect, 27*(2), 169–190. https://doi.org/10.1016/S0145-2134(02)00541-0

Bernstein, E. M., & Putnam, F. W. (1986). Development, reliability, and validity of a dissociation scale. *Journal of Nervous and Mental Disease, 174*(12), 727–735. https://doi.org/10.1097/00005053-198612000-00004

Bigras, N., Godbout, N., Hébert, M., Runtz, M., & Daspe, M. È. (2015). Identity and relatedness as mediators between child emotional abuse and adult couple adjustment in women. *Child Abuse & Neglect, 50*, 85–93. https://doi.org/10.1016/j.chiabu.2015.07.009

Birmes, P., Carreras, D., Ducassé, J. L., Charlet, J. P., Warner, B. A., Lauque, D., & Schmitt, L. (2001). Peritraumatic dissociation, acute stress, and early post-traumatic stress disorder in victims of general crime. *Canadian Journal of Psychiatry, 46*(7), 649–651. https://doi.org/10.1177/070674370104600711

Black, M. C., Basile, K. C., Breiding, M. J., Smith, S. G., Walters, M. L., Merrick, M. T., Chen, J., & Stevens, M. R. (2011). *The National Intimate Partner and Sexual Violence Survey (NISVS): 2010 summary report.* National Center for Injury Prevention and Control, Centers for Disease Control and Prevention.

Blackmore, E. R., Côté-Arsenault, D., Tang, W., Glover, V., Evans, J., Golding, J., & O'Connor, T. G. (2011). Previous prenatal loss as a predictor of perinatal depression and anxiety. *The British Journal of Psychiatry, 198*(5), 373–378. https://doi.org/10.1192/bjp.bp.110.083105

Blake, D. D., Weathers, F. W., Nagy, L. M., Kaloupek, D. G., Gusman, F. D., Charney, D. S., & Keane, T. M. (1995). The development of a clinician-administered PTSD scale. *Journal of Traumatic Stress, 8*(1), 75–90. https://doi.org/10.1002/jts.2490080106

Blake, D. D., Weathers, F. W., Nagy, L. M., Kaloupek, D. G., Klauminzer, G., Charney, D. S., & Keane, T. M. (1990). A clinician rating scale for assessing current and lifetime PTSD: The CAPS-1. *Behavior Therapist, 13*, 187–188.

Blanchard, E. B., & Hickling, E. J. (2004). *After the crash: Psychological assessment and treatment of motor vehicle survivors* (2nd ed.). American Psychological Association. https://doi.org/10.1037/10676-000

Blanchard, E. B., Hickling, E. J., Devineni, T., Veazey, C. H., Galovski, T. E., Mundy, E., Malta, L. S., & Buckley, T. C. (2003). A controlled evaluation of cognitive behavioural therapy for posttraumatic stress in motor vehicle accident survivors. *Behaviour Research and Therapy, 41*(1), 79–96. https://doi.org/10.1016/S0005-7967(01)00131-0

Blanco, C., Alegría, A. A., Petry, N. M., Grant, J. E., Simpson, H. B., Liu, S. M., Grant, B. F., & Hasin, D. S. (2010). Prevalence and correlates of fire-setting in the United States: Results from the National Epidemiologic Survey on Alcohol and Related Conditions (NESARC). *The Journal of Clinical Psychiatry, 71*(9), 1218–1225. https://doi.org/10.4088/JCP.08m04812gry

Blevins, C. A., Weathers, F. W., Davis, M. T., Witte, T. K., & Domino, J. L. (2015). The Posttraumatic Stress Disorder Checklist for DSM-5 (PCL-5): Development and initial psychometric evaluation. *Journal of Traumatic Stress, 28*(6), 489–498. https://doi.org/10.1002/jts.22059

Blohm, F., Fridén, B., & Milsom, I. (2008). A prospective longitudinal population-based study of clinical miscarriage in an urban Swedish population. *BJOG, 115*(2), 176–182. https://doi.org/10.1111/j.1471-0528.2007.01426.x

Boelen, P. A., Olff, M., & Smid, G. E. (2019). Traumatic loss: Mental health consequences and implications for treatment and prevention. *European Journal of Psychotraumatology, 10*(1), 1591331. https://doi.org/10.1080/20008198.2019.1591331

Bovin, M. J., Kimerling, R., Weathers, F. W., Prins, A., Marx, B. P., Post, E. P., & Schnurr, P. P. (2021). Diagnostic accuracy and acceptability of the Primary Care Posttraumatic Stress Disorder Screen for the *Diagnostic and Statistical Manual of Mental Disorders (Fifth Edition)* among US Veterans. *JAMA Network Open, 4*(2), e2036733. https://doi.org/10.1001/jamanetworkopen.2020.36733

Bovin, M. J., Marx, B. P., Weathers, F. W., Gallagher, M. W., Rodriguez, P., Schnurr, P. P., & Keane, T. M. (2016). Psychometric properties of the PTSD Checklist for *Diagnostic and Statistical Manual of Mental Disorders-Fifth Edition* (PCL-5) in veterans. *Psychological Assessment, 28*(11), 1379–1391. https://doi.org/10.1037/pas0000254

Bovin, M. J., Schneiderman, A., Bernhard, P. A., Maguen, S., Hoffmire, C. A., Blosnich, J. R., Smith, B. N., Kulka, R., & Vogt, D. (2023). Development and validation of a brief warfare exposure measure among U.S. Iraq and Afghanistan war veterans: The Deployment Risk and Resilience Inventory-2 Warfare Exposure—Short Form (DRRI-2 WE-SF). *Psychological Trauma: Theory, Research, Practice, and Policy, 15*(8), 1248–1258. https://doi.org/10.1037/tra0001282

Brabin, P. J., & Berah, E. F. (1995). Dredging up past traumas: Harmful or helpful? *Psychiatry, Psychology, and Law, 2*(2), 165–171. https://doi.org/10.1080/13218719509524863

Brand, B. L. (2024). *The concise guide to the assessment and treatment of trauma-related dissociation.* American Psychological Association. https://doi.org/10.1037/0000386-000

Brand, B. L., Armstrong, J., & Loewenstein, R. (2006). Psychological assessment of patients with dissociative identity disorder. *The Psychiatric Clinics of North America, 29*, 145–168. https://doi.org/10.1016/j.psc.2005.10.014

Brand, B. L., & Chasson, G. S. (2015). Distinguishing simulated from genuine dissociative identity disorder on the MMPI-2. *Psychological Trauma: Theory, Research, Practice, and Policy, 7*(1), 93–101. https://doi.org/10.1037/a0035181

Brand, B. L., Chasson, G. S., Palermo, C. A., Donato, F., Rhodes, K., & Voorhees, E. F. (2016). MMPI-2 item endorsements in dissociative identity disorder vs. simulators. *Journal of the American Academy of Psychiatry and the Law, 44*(1), 63–72.

Brand, B. L., Dalenberg, C. J., Frewen, P. A., Loewenstein, R. J., Schielke, H. J., Brams, J. S., & Spiegel, D. (2018). Trauma-related dissociation is no fantasy: Addressing the errors of omission and commission in Merckelbach and Patihis (2018). *Psychological Injury and Law, 11*(4), 377–393. https://doi.org/10.1007/s12207-018-9336-8

Brand, B. L., & Lanius, R. A. (2014). Chronic complex dissociative disorders and borderline personality disorder: Disorders of emotion dysregulation? *Borderline Personality Disorder and Emotion Dysregulation, 1*(1), 13. https://doi.org/10.1186/2051-6673-1-13

Brand, B. L., Schielke, H. J., Schiavone, F., & Lanius, R. A. (2022). *Finding solid ground: Overcoming obstacles in trauma treatment.* Oxford University Press. https://doi.org/10.1093/med-psych/9780190636081.001.0001

Brave Heart, M. Y., & DeBruyn, L. M. (1998). The American Indian Holocaust: Healing historical unresolved grief. *American Indian and Alaska Native Mental Health Research, 8*(2), 56–78.

Bremner, J. D., Krystal, J. H., Putnam, F. W., Southwick, S. M., Marmar, C., Charney, D. S., & Mazure, C. M. (1998). Measurement of dissociative states with the Clinician-Administered Dissociative States Scale (CADSS). *Journal of Traumatic Stress, 11*(1), 125–136. https://doi.org/10.1023/A:1024465317902

Breslau, N., & Davis, G. C. (1992). Posttraumatic stress disorder in an urban population of young adults: Risk factors for chronicity. *The American Journal of Psychiatry, 149*(5), 671–675. https://doi.org/10.1176/ajp.149.5.671

Brewin, C. R., Andrews, B., & Rose, S. (2000). Fear, helplessness, and horror in posttraumatic stress disorder: Investigating DSM-IV Criterion A2 in victims of violent crime. *Journal of Traumatic Stress, 13*(3), 499–509. https://doi.org/10.1023/A:1007741526169

Brewin, C. R., Andrews, B., Rose, S., & Kirk, M. (1999). Acute stress disorder and posttraumatic stress disorder in victims of violent crime. *The American Journal of Psychiatry, 156*(3), 360–366. https://doi.org/10.1176/ajp.156.3.360

Bridgland, V. M. E., Moeck, E. K., Green, D. M., Swain, T. L., Nayda, D. M., Matson, L. A., Hutchison, N. P., & Takarangi, M. K. T. (2021). Why the COVID-19 pandemic is a traumatic stressor. *PLoS One, 16*(1), e0240146. https://doi.org/10.1371/journal.pone.0240146

Briere, J. (1992). Medical symptoms, health risk, and history of childhood sexual abuse. *Mayo Clinic Proceedings, 67*(6), 603–604. https://doi.org/10.1016/S0025-6196(12)60471-6

Briere, J. (1995). *Trauma Symptom Inventory (TSI)*. Psychological Assessment Resources.

Briere, J. (1996). *Trauma Symptom Checklist for Children (TSCC)*. Psychological Assessment Resources.

Briere, J. (2000a). *Cognitive Distortions Scale (CDS)*. Psychological Assessment Resources.

Briere, J. (2000b). *Inventory of Altered Self Capacities (IASC)*. Psychological Assessment Resources.

Briere, J. (2001). *Detailed Assessment of Posttraumatic Stress (DAPS)*. Psychological Assessment Resources.

Briere, J. (2002). *Multiscale Dissociation Inventory*. Psychological Assessment Resources.

Briere, J. (2004). *Psychological assessment of adult posttraumatic states: Phenomenology, diagnosis, and measurement* (2nd ed.). American Psychological Association. https://doi.org/10.1037/10809-000

Briere, J. (2011). *Trauma Symptom Inventory-2 (TSI-2)*. Psychological Assessment Resources.

Briere, J. (2013). *PTSD and Suicide Screener (PSS) professional manual*. Psychological Assessment Resources.

Briere, J. (2019). *Treating risky and compulsive behavior in trauma survivors*. Guilford Press.

Briere, J. (2023). *Social Discrimination and Maltreatment Scale–Short Form* [Unpublished psychological test]. Keck School of Medicine, University of Southern California.

Briere, J. (2024). *Broadband trauma/adversity review (BTAR)* [Unpublished psychological test]. Keck School of Medicine, University of Southern California.

Briere, J., Agee, E., & Dietrich, A. (2016). Cumulative trauma and current posttraumatic stress disorder status in general population and inmate samples. *Psychological Trauma: Theory, Research, Practice, and Policy, 8*(4), 439–446. https://doi.org/10.1037/tra0000107

Briere, J., Dias, C. P., Semple, R. J., Scott, C., Bigras, N., & Godbout, N. (2017). Acute stress symptoms in seriously injured patients: Precipitating versus cumulative trauma and the contribution of peritraumatic distress. *Journal of Traumatic Stress, 30*(4), 381–388. https://doi.org/10.1002/jts.22200

Briere, J., & Eadie, E. M. (2016). Compensatory self-injury: Posttraumatic stress, depression, and the role of dissociation. *Psychological Trauma: Theory, Research, and Practice, 8*(5), 618–625. https://doi.org/10.1037/tra0000139

Briere, J., & Elliott, D. (2000). Prevalence, characteristics, and long-term sequelae of natural disaster exposure in the general population. *Journal of Traumatic Stress, 13*(4), 661–679. https://doi.org/10.1023/A:1007814301369

Briere, J., & Elliott, D. M. (2003). Prevalence and psychological sequelae of self-reported childhood physical and sexual abuse in a general population sample of men and women. *Child Abuse & Neglect, 27*(10), 1205–1222. https://doi.org/10.1016/j.chiabu.2003.09.008

Briere, J., Godbout, N., & Runtz, M. (2012). The Psychological Maltreatment Review (PMR): Initial reliability and association with insecure attachment in adults. *Journal of Aggression, Maltreatment & Trauma, 21*(3), 300–320. https://doi.org/10.1080/10926771.2012.659801

Briere, J., Goldin, J. N., & Rodriguez, M. M. (2003). *Detailed Assessment of Posttraumatic Stress Interpretive Report for Windows® (DAPS-IR)*. Psychological Assessment Resources.

Briere, J., Kaltman, S., & Green, B. L. (2008). Accumulated childhood trauma and symptom complexity. *Journal of Traumatic Stress, 21*(2), 223–226. https://doi.org/10.1002/jts.20317

Briere, J., Kwon, O., Semple, R., & Godbout, N. (2019). Recent suicidal ideation and behavior in the general population: The role of depression, posttraumatic stress, and reactive avoidance. *Journal of Nervous and Mental Disease, 207*(5), 320–325. https://doi.org/10.1097/NMD.0000000000000976

Briere, J., & Lanktree, C. B. (2012). *Treating complex trauma in adolescents and young adults.* https://doi.org/10.4135/9781452240497

Briere, J., Lanktree, C. B., & Escott, A. (2020). *Trauma teletherapy for youth in the era of the COVID-19 pandemic: Adapting evidence-based treatment approaches.* University of Southern California Adolescent Trauma Training Center, National Child Traumatic Stress Network, Substance Abuse and Mental Health Services Administration.

Briere, J., Madni, L. A., & Godbout, N. (2016). Recent suicidality in the general population: Multivariate association with childhood maltreatment and adult victimization. *Journal of Interpersonal Violence, 31*(18), 3063–3079. https://doi.org/10.1177/0886260515584339

Briere, J., & Rickards, S. (2007). Self-awareness, affect regulation, and relatedness: Differential sequels of childhood versus adult victimization experiences. *Journal of Nervous and Mental Disease, 195*(6), 497–503. https://doi.org/10.1097/NMD.0b013e31803044e2

Briere, J., & Runtz, M. (2002). The Inventory of Altered Self-Capacities (IASC): A standardized measure of identity, affect regulation, and relationship disturbance. *Assessment, 9*(3), 230–239. https://doi.org/10.1177/1073191102009003002

Briere, J., & Runtz, M. (2024). Police in the rearview mirror: Social marginalization, trauma, and fear of being killed. *American Journal of Orthopsychiatry, 94*(1), 15–22. https://psycnet.apa.org/doi/10.1037/ort0000700

Briere, J., Runtz, M., Eadie, E., Bigras, N., & Godbout, N. (2017). Disengaged parenting: Structural equation modeling with child abuse, insecure attachment, and adult symptomatology. *Child Abuse & Neglect, 67*, 260–270. https://doi.org/10.1016/j.chiabu.2017.02.036

Briere, J., Runtz, M., Eadie, E. M., Bigras, N., & Godbout, N. (2019). The Disorganized Response Scale: Construct validity of a potential self-report measure of disorganized attachment. *Psychological Trauma: Theory, Research, Practice, and Policy, 11*(5), 486–494. https://doi.org/10.1037/tra0000396

Briere, J., Runtz, M., Rassart, C.-A., Rodd, K., & Godbout, N. (2020). Sexual assault trauma: Does prior childhood maltreatment increase the risk and exacerbate the outcome? *Child Abuse & Neglect, 103*, 104421. https://doi.org/10.1016/j.chiabu.2020.104421

Briere, J., Runtz, M., & Rodd, K. (2024). Child and adolescent exposure to sexual harassment: Relationship to gender, contact sexual abuse, and adult psychological symptoms. *Journal of Interpersonal Violence, 39*(13–14), 2981–2996. https://doi.org/10.1177/08862605231225524

Briere, J., Runtz, M., & Rodd, K. (2025). Social maltreatment as trauma: Posttraumatic correlates of a new measure of exposure to sexism, racism, and cisheterosexism. *Psychological Trauma: Theory, Research, Practice, and Policy, 17*(2), 387–395. https://doi.org/10.1037/tra0001636

Briere, J., Runtz, M. R., Villenueve, E., & Godbout, N. (2024). Social maltreatment and symptomatology: Validating the Social Discrimination and Maltreatment Scale–Short Form (SDMS-SF) in a diverse sample. *Journal of Interpersonal Violence*. Advance online publication. https://doi.org/10.1177/08862605241301791

Briere, J., & Scott, C. (2007). Assessment of trauma symptoms in eating-disordered populations. *Eating Disorders: The Journal of Treatment & Prevention, 15*(4), 347–358. https://doi.org/10.1080/10640260701454360

Briere, J., & Scott, C. (2014). *Principles of trauma therapy: A guide to symptoms, evaluation, and treatment* (2nd ed., DSM-5 update). Sage.

Briere, J., & Scott, C. (2015). Complex trauma in adolescents and adults: Effects and treatment. *The Psychiatric Clinics of North America, 38*(3), 515–527. https://doi.org/10.1016/j.psc.2015.05.004

Briere, J., Scott, C., & Weathers, F. (2005). Peritraumatic and persistent dissociation in the presumed etiology of PTSD. *The American Journal of Psychiatry, 162*(12), 2295–2301. https://doi.org/10.1176/appi.ajp.162.12.2295

Briere, J., Weathers, F. W., & Runtz, M. (2005). Is dissociation a multidimensional construct? Data from the Multiscale Dissociation Inventory. *Journal of Traumatic Stress, 18*(3), 221–231. https://doi.org/10.1002/jts.20024

Briere, J., & Zaidi, L. Y. (1989). Sexual abuse histories and sequelae in female psychiatric emergency room patients. *The American Journal of Psychiatry, 146*(12), 1602–1606. https://doi.org/10.1176/ajp.146.12.1602

Briggs, E. C., Amaya-Jackson, L., Putnam, K., & Putnam, F. W. (2021). All adverse childhood experiences are not equal: The contribution of synergy to adverse childhood experience scores. *The American Psychologist, 76*(2), 243–252. https://doi.org/10.1037/amp0000768

Brockell, G. (2021, March 18). The long, ugly history of anti-Asian racism and violence in the U.S. *The Washington Post*. https://www.washingtonpost.com/history/2021/03/18/history-anti-asian-violence-racism/

Brown, E. J., & Heimberg, R. G. (2001). Effects of writing about rape: Evaluating Pennebaker's paradigm with a severe trauma. *Journal of Traumatic Stress, 14*(4), 781–790. https://doi.org/10.1023/A:1013098307063

Brown, P. J., & Wolfe, J. (1994). Substance abuse and post-traumatic stress disorder comorbidity. *Drug and Alcohol Dependence, 35*(1), 51–59. https://doi.org/10.1016/0376-8716(94)90110-4

Brown, T. A., & Barlow, D. H. (2014). *Anxiety and Related Disorders Interview Schedule for DSM-5 (ADIS-5)–Adult Version.* Oxford University Press.

Brown, T. A., Campbell, L. A., Lehman, C. L., Grisham, J. R., & Mancill, R. B. (2001). Current and lifetime comorbidity of the *DSM-IV* anxiety and mood disorders in a large clinical sample. *Journal of Abnormal Psychology, 110*(4), 585–599. https://doi.org/10.1037/0021-843X.110.4.585

Brown, T. A., DiNardo, P. A., & Barlow, D. H. (1994). *Anxiety Disorders Interview Schedule for DSM-IV (ADIS-4).* Psychological Corporation.

Bryant, R. A. (2016). *Acute stress disorder: What it is and how to treat it.* Guilford Press.

Bryant, R. A., Creamer, M., O'Donnell, M., Silove, D., McFarlane, A. C., & Forbes, D. (2015). A comparison of the capacity of *DSM-IV* and *DSM-5* acute stress disorder definitions to predict posttraumatic stress disorder and related disorders. *The Journal of Clinical Psychiatry, 76*(4), 391–397. https://doi.org/10.4088/JCP.13m08731

Bryant, R. A., & Harvey, A. G. (1999). Acute stress disorder following motor vehicle accidents. In E. J. Hickling & L. B. Blanchard (Eds.), *The international handbook of road traffic accidents and psychological trauma: Current understanding, treatment and law* (pp. 29–42). Elsevier Science.

Bryant, R. A., Harvey, A. G., Dang, S. T., & Sackville, T. (1998). Assessing acute stress disorder: Psychometric properties of a structured clinical interview. *Psychological Assessment, 10*(3), 215–220. https://doi.org/10.1037/1040-3590.10.3.215

Bryant, R. A., Moulds, M. L., & Guthrie, R. M. (2000). Acute Stress Disorder Scale: A self-report measure of acute stress disorder. *Psychological Assessment, 12*(1), 61–68. https://doi.org/10.1037/1040-3590.12.1.61

Bub, K., & Lommen, M. J. J. (2017). The role of guilt in posttraumatic stress disorder. *European Journal of Psychotraumatology, 8*(1), 1407202. https://doi.org/10.1080/20008198.2017.1407202

Bureau, J.-F., Martin, J., & Lyons-Ruth, K. (2010). Attachment dysregulation as hidden trauma in infancy: Early stress, maternal buffering, and psychiatric morbidity in young adulthood. In R. A. Lanius, E. Vermetten, & C. Pain (Eds.), *The impact of early life trauma on health and disease: The hidden epidemic* (pp. 48–56). Cambridge University Press.

Busby, D. M., Glenn, E., Steggell, G. L., & Adamson, D. W. (1993). Treatment issues for survivors of physical and sexual abuse. *Journal of Marital and Family Therapy, 19*(4), 377–392. https://doi.org/10.1111/j.1752-0606.1993.tb01000.x

Buswell, G., Haime, Z., Lloyd-Evans, B., & Billings, J. (2021). A systematic review of PTSD to the experience of psychosis: Prevalence and associated factors. *BMC Psychiatry, 21*(1), 9. https://doi.org/10.1186/s12888-020-02999-x

Butcher, J. N., Dahlstrom, W. G., Graham, J. R., Tellegen, A., & Kaemmer, B. (1989). *Minnesota Multiphasic Personality Inventory (MMPI-2): Manual for administration and scoring.* University of Minnesota Press.

Butler, B., & Welch, J. (2009). Drug-facilitated sexual assault. *Canadian Medical Association Journal, 180*(5), 493–494. https://doi.org/10.1503/cmaj.090006

Callaway, K. L., & Spates, R. C. (2016). Moral injury in military members and veterans. In *Oxford handbook topics in psychology.* Oxford University Press. https://doi.org/10.1093/oxfordhb/9780199935291.013.69

Canan, F., & North, C. S. (2019). Dissociation and disasters: A systematic review. *World Journal of Psychiatry, 9*(6), 83–98. https://doi.org/10.5498/wjp.v9.i6.83

Cantor, J. (2011). New MRI studies support the Blanchard typology of male-to-female transsexualism. *Archives of Sexual Behavior, 40,* 863–864. https://doi.org/10.1007/s10508-011-9805-6

Cardeña, E., & Carlson, E. (2011). Acute stress disorder revisited. *Annual Review of Clinical Psychology, 7*(1), 245–267. https://doi.org/10.1146/annurev-clinpsy-032210-104502

Cardeña, E., Koopman, C., Classen, C., & Spiegel, D. (1996). Review of the Stanford Acute Stress Reaction Questionnaire. In B. H. Stamm (Ed.), *Measurement of stress, trauma and adaptation* (pp. 293–297). Sidran Press.

Cardeña, E., Koopman, C., Classen, C., Waelde, L. C., & Spiegel, D. (2000). Psychometric properties of the Stanford Acute Stress Reaction Questionnaire (SASRQ): A valid and reliable measure of acute stress. *Journal of Traumatic Stress, 13*(4), 719–734. https://doi.org/10.1023/A:1007822603186

Carleton, R. N., Peluso, D. L., Collimore, K. C., & Asmundson, G. J. G. (2011). Social anxiety and posttraumatic stress symptoms: The impact of distressing social events. *Journal of Anxiety Disorders, 25*(1), 49–57. https://doi.org/10.1016/j.janxdis.2010.08.002

Carlozzi, N. E., & Long, P. J. (2008). Reliability and validity of the SCL-90-R PTSD subscale. *Journal of Interpersonal Violence, 23*(9), 1162–1176. https://doi.org/10.1177/0886260508314295

Carlson, E. B. (1997). *Trauma assessments: A clinician's guide.* Guilford Press.

Carlson, E. B. (2001). Psychometric study of a brief screen for PTSD: Assessing the impact of multiple traumatic events. *Assessment, 8*(4), 431–441. https://doi.org/10.1177/107319110100800408

Carlson, E. B., & Dalenberg, C. J. (2000). A conceptual framework for the impact of traumatic experiences. *Trauma, Violence, and Abuse: A Review Journal, 1,* 4–28.

Carlson, E. B., & Putnam, F. W. (1993). An update on the Dissociative Experience Scale. *Dissociation, 6*(1), 16–27.

Carlson, E. B., Smith, S. R., & Dalenberg, C. J. (2013). Can sudden, severe emotional loss be a traumatic stressor? *Journal of Trauma & Dissociation, 14*(5), 519–528. https://doi.org/10.1080/15299732.2013.773475

Carlson, E. B., Smith, S. R., Palmieri, P. A., Dalenberg, C., Ruzek, J. I., Kimerling, R., Burling, T. A., & Spain, D. A. (2011). Development and validation of a brief self-report measure of trauma exposure: The Trauma History Screen. *Psychological Assessment, 23*(2), 463–477. https://doi.org/10.1037/a0022294

Carter, R. T., Mazzula, S., Victoria, R., Vazquez, R., Hall, S., Smith, S., Sant-Barket, S., Forsyth, J., Bazelais, K., & Williams, B. (2013). Initial development of the Race-Based Traumatic Stress Symptom Scale: Assessing the emotional impact of racism. *Psychological Trauma: Theory, Research, Practice, and Policy, 5*(1), 1–9. https://doi.org/10.1037/a0025911

Centers for Disease Control and Prevention. (2024). *Health Insurance Portability and Accountability Act (HIPPA) of 1996.* https://www.cdc.gov/phlp/php/resources/health-insurance-portability-and-accountability-act-of-1996-hipaa.html

Charlton, J. P., & Danforth, I. D. W. (2007). Distinguishing addiction and high engagement in the context of online game playing. *Computers in Human Behavior, 23*(3), 1531–1548. https://doi.org/10.1016/j.chb.2005.07.002

Chilcoat, H. D., & Breslau, N. (1998). Investigations of causal pathways between PTSD and drug use disorders. *Addictive Behaviors, 23*(6), 827–840. https://doi.org/10.1016/S0306-4603(98)00069-0

Choca, J. P., Shanley, L. A., & Van Denburg, E. (1992). *Interpretive guide to the Millon Clinical Multiaxial Inventory.* American Psychological Association. https://doi.org/10.1037/11094-000

Cloitre, M., Garvert, D. W., Weiss, B., Carlson, E. B., & Bryant, R. A. (2014). Distinguishing PTSD, complex PTSD, and borderline personality disorder: A latent class analysis. *European Journal of Psychotraumatology, 5*(1), 25097. https://doi.org/10.3402/ejpt.v5.25097

Cloitre, M., Shevlin, M., Brewin, C. R., Bisson, J. I., Roberts, N. P., Maercker, A., Karatzias, T., & Hyland, P. (2018). The International Trauma Questionnaire: Development of a self-report measure of ICD-11 PTSD and complex PTSD. *Acta Psychiatrica Scandinavica, 138*(6), 536–546. https://doi.org/10.1111/acps.12956

Cloitre, M., Stolbach, B., & Herman, J. (2009). A developmental approach to complex PTSD: Childhood and adult cumulative trauma as predictors of symptom complexity. *Journal of Traumatic Stress, 22*, 399–408.

Cloitre, M., Stolbach, B. C., Herman, J. L., van der Kolk, B., Pynoos, R., Wang, J., & Petkova, E. (2009). A developmental approach to complex PTSD: Childhood and adult cumulative trauma as predictors of symptom complexity. *Journal of Traumatic Stress, 22*(5), 399–408. https://doi.org/10.1002/jts.20444

Committee on the Assessment of Ongoing Efforts in the Treatment of Post-traumatic Stress Disorder, Board on the Health of Select Populations, & Institute of Medicine. (2014). *Treatment for posttraumatic stress disorder in military and veteran populations: Final assessment.* National Academies Press.

Compean, E., & Hamner, M. (2019). Posttraumatic stress disorder with secondary psychotic features (PTSD-SP): Diagnostic and treatment challenges. *Progress in Neuro-Psychopharmacology & Biological Psychiatry, 88*, 265–275. https://doi.org/10.1016/j.pnpbp.2018.08.001

Connor, K. M., & Davidson, J. R. (2001). SPRINT: A brief global assessment of post-traumatic stress disorder. *International Clinical Psychopharmacology, 16*(5), 279–284. https://doi.org/10.1097/00004850-200109000-00005

Cook, A., Spinazzola, J., Ford, J., Lanktree, C., Blaustein, M., Cloitre, M., DeRosa, R., Hubbard, R., Kagan, R., Liautaurd, J., Mallah, K, Olafson, E., & van der Kolk, B. (2005). Complex trauma in children and adolescents. *Psychiatric Annals, 35*(5), 390–398. https://doi.org/10.3928/00485713-20050501-05

Cougle, J. R., Feldner, M. T., Keough, M. E., Hawkins, K. A., & Fitch, K. E. (2010). Comorbid panic attacks among individuals with posttraumatic stress disorder: Associations with traumatic event exposure history, symptoms, and impairment. *Journal of Anxiety Disorders, 24*(2), 183–188. https://doi.org/10.1016/j.janxdis.2009.10.006

Courtois, C. (1995). Assessment and diagnosis. In C. Classen (Ed.), *Treating women molested in childhood* (pp. 1–54). Jossey-Bass.

Courtois, C. A. (1999). *Recollections of sexual abuse: Treatment principles and guidelines*. W. W. Norton & Company.

Courtois, C. A. (2004). Complex trauma, complex reactions: Assessment and treatment. *Psychotherapy: Theory, Research, & Practice, 41*(4), 412–425. https://doi.org/10.1037/0033-3204.41.4.412

Courtois, C. A., & Ford, J. D. (Eds.). (2009). *Treating complex traumatic stress disorders: An evidence-based guide*. Guilford Press.

Craig, A., Tran, Y., Guest, R., Gopinath, B., Jagnoor, J., Bryant, R. A., Collie, A., Tate, R., Kenardy, J., Middleton, J. W., & Cameron, I. (2016). Psychological impact of injuries sustained in motor vehicle crashes: Systematic review and meta-analysis. *BMJ Open, 6*(9), e011993. https://doi.org/10.1136/bmjopen-2016-011993

Craig, R. J., & Olson, R. (1997). Assessing PTSD with the Millon Clinical Multiaxial Inventory-III. *Journal of Clinical Psychology, 53*(8), 943–952. https://doi.org/10.1002/(SICI)1097-4679(199712)53:8<943::AID-JCLP20>3.0.CO;2-J

Creamer, M., Bell, R., & Failla, S. (2003). Psychometric properties of the Impact of Event Scale–Revised. *Behaviour Research and Therapy, 41*(12), 1489–1496. https://doi.org/10.1016/j.brat.2003.07.010

Currier, G. W., & Briere, J. (2000). Trauma orientation and detection of violence histories in the psychiatric emergency service. *Journal of Nervous and Mental Disease, 188*(9), 622–624. https://doi.org/10.1097/00005053-200009000-00011

Cyr, G., Godbout, N., Cloitre, M., & Bélanger, C. (2022). Distinguishing among symptoms of posttraumatic stress disorder, complex posttraumatic stress disorder, and borderline personality disorder in a community sample of women. *Journal of Traumatic Stress, 35*(1), 186–196. https://doi.org/10.1002/jts.22719

Dalenberg, C. J., Brand, B. L., Gleaves, D. H., Dorahy, M. J., Loewenstein, R. J., Cardeña, E., Frewen, P. A., Carlson, E. B., & Spiegel, D. (2012). Evaluation of the evidence for the trauma and fantasy models of dissociation. *Psychological Bulletin, 138*(3), 550–588. https://doi.org/10.1037/a0027447

Dalenberg, C. J., Brand, B. L., Loewenstein, R. J., Frewen, P. A., & Spiegel, D. (2020). Inviting scientific discourse on traumatic dissociation: Progress made and obstacles to further resolution. *Psychological Injury and Law, 13*(2), 135–154. https://doi.org/10.1007/s12207-020-09376-9

Dalenberg, C. J., & Palesh, O. G. (2004). Relationship between child abuse history, trauma, and dissociation in Russian college students. *Child Abuse & Neglect, 28*(4), 461–474. https://doi.org/10.1016/j.chiabu.2003.11.020

D'Alessandro, A. M., Ritchie, K., McCabe, R. E., Lanius, R. A., Heber, A., Smith, P., Malain, A., Schielke, H., O'Connor, C., Hosseiny, F., Rodrigues, S., & McKinnon, M. C. (2022). Healthcare workers and COVID-19-related moral injury: An interpersonally-focused approach informed by PTSD. *Frontiers in Psychiatry, 12*, 784523. https://doi.org/10.3389/fpsyt.2021.784523

David, D., Kutcher, G. S., Jackson, E. I., & Mellman, T. A. (1999). Psychotic symptoms in combat-related posttraumatic stress disorder. *The Journal of Clinical Psychiatry, 60*(1), 29–32. https://doi.org/10.4088/JCP.v60n0106

Davidson, J. (2002). *SPAN addendum to DTS manual*. Multi-Health Systems Inc.

Davidson, J., Smith, R., & Kudler, H. (1989). Validity and reliability of the *DSM-III* criteria for posttraumatic stress disorder: Experience with a structured interview. *Journal of Nervous and Mental Disease, 177*, 336–341.

Davidson, J. R. T., Book, S. W., Colket, J. T., Tupler, L. A., Roth, S., David, D., Hertzberg, M., Mellman, T., Beckham, J. C., Smith, R. D., Davison, R. M., Katz, R., & Feldman, M. E. (1997). Assessment of a new self-rating scale for post-traumatic stress disorder. *Psychological Medicine, 27*(1), 153–160. https://doi.org/10.1017/S0033291796004229

Davidson, J. R. T., Tharwani, H. M., & Connor, K. M. (2002). Davidson Trauma Scale (DTS): Normative scores in the general population and effect sizes in placebo-controlled SSRI trials. *Depression and Anxiety, 15*(2), 75–78. https://doi.org/10.1002/da.10021

de Jong, J. T. V. M., Komproe, I. H., Van Ommeren, M., El Masri, M., Araya, M., Khaled, N., van De Put, W., & Somasundaram, D. (2001). Lifetime events and posttraumatic stress disorder in 4 postconflict settings. *JAMA, 286*(5), 555–562. https://doi.org/10.1001/jama.286.5.555

Decker, M. L., Littleton, H., & Edwards, K. M. (2018). An updated review of the literature on LGBTQ+ intimate partner violence. *Current Sexual Health Reports, 10*(4), 265–272. https://doi.org/10.1007/s11930-018-0173-2

DeGruy, J. (2017). *Post traumatic slave syndrome: America's legacy of enduring injury and healing* (Rev. ed.). Joy DeGruy Publications Inc.

Dell, P. F. (2006). The multidimensional inventory of dissociation (MID): A comprehensive measure of pathological dissociation. *Journal of Trauma & Dissociation, 7*(2), 77–106. https://doi.org/10.1300/J229v07n02_06

Denton, R., Frogley, C., Jackson, S., John, M., & Querstret, D. (2017). The assessment of developmental trauma in children and adolescents: A systematic review.

Clinical Child Psychology and Psychiatry, 22(2), 260–287. https://doi.org/10.1177/1359104516631607

Derogatis, L. R. (1993). *BSI brief symptom inventory: Administration, scoring, and procedures manual* (4th ed.). National Computer Systems.

Derogatis, L. R. (1994). *SCL-90-R: Administration, scoring and procedures manual* (3rd ed.). National Computer Systems.

Derogatis, L. R., Lipman, R. S., Rickels, K., Uhlenhuth, E. H., & Covi, L. (1974). The Hopkins Symptom Checklist (HSCL): A self-report symptom inventory. *Behavioral Science, 19*(1), 1–15. https://doi.org/10.1002/bs.3830190102

de Vries, B., van Busschbach, J. T., van der Stouwe, E. C. D., Aleman, A., van Dijk, J. J. Lysaker, P. H., Arends, J., Nijman, S. A., & Pijnenborg, G.M. (2019). Prevalence rate and risk factors of victimization in adult patients with a psychotic disorder: A systematic review and meta-analysis. *Schizophrenia Bulletin, 45*(1), 114–126. https://doi.org/10.1093/schbul/sby020

De Zulueta, F. I. S. (1998). Human violence: A treatable epidemic. *Medicine, Conflict, and Survival, 14*(1), 46–55. https://doi.org/10.1080/13623699808409371

Diamantopoulos, A., Sarstedt, M., Fuchs, C., Wilczynski, P., & Kaiser, S. (2012). Guidelines for choosing between multi-item and single-item scales for construct measurement: A predictive validity perspective. *Journal of the Academy of Marketing Science, 40*(3), 434–449. https://doi.org/10.1007/s11747-011-0300-3

Dichter, M. E., Thomas, K. A., Crits-Christoph, P., Ogden, S. N., & Rhodes, K. V. (2018). Coercive control in intimate partner violence: Relationship with women's experience of violence, use of violence, and danger. *Psychology of Violence, 8*(5), 596–604. https://doi.org/10.1037/vio0000158

DiGrande, L., Neria, Y., Brackbill, R. M., Pulliam, P., & Galea, S. (2011). Long-term posttraumatic stress symptoms among 3,271 civilian survivors of the September 11, 2001, terrorist attacks on the World Trade Center. *American Journal of Epidemiology, 173*(3), 271–281. https://doi.org/10.1093/aje/kwq372

Dietrich, A. M. (2003). Characteristics of child maltreatment, psychological dissociation, and somatoform dissociation of Canadian inmates. *Journal of Trauma and Dissociation, 4*, 81–100.

Dong, X., Chen, R., Chang, E. S., & Simon, M. (2013). Elder abuse and psychological well-being: A systematic review and implications for research and policy—A mini review. *Gerontology, 59*(2), 132–142. https://doi.org/10.1159/000341652

Drescher, K. D., Foy, D. W., Kelly, C., Leshner, A., Schutz, K., & Litz, B. (2011). An exploration of the viability and usefulness of the construct of moral injury in war veterans. *Traumatology, 17*(1), 8–13. https://doi.org/10.1177/1534765610395615

Driessen, M., Herrmann, J., Stahl, K., Zwaan, M., Meier, S., Hill, A., Osterheider, M., & Petersen, D. (2000). Magnetic resonance imaging volumes of the hippocampus and the amygdala in women with borderline personality disorder and early traumatization. *Archives of General Psychiatry, 57*(12), 1115–1122. https://doi.org/10.1001/archpsyc.57.12.1115

Drury, P., Calhoun, P. S., Boggs, C., Araujo, G., Dennis, M. F., & Beckham, J. C. (2009). Influences of comorbid disorders on Personality Assessment Inventory profiles in women with posttraumatic stress disorder. *Journal of Psychopathology and Behavioral Assessment, 31*(2), 119–128. https://doi.org/10.1007/s10862-008-9101-5

Dube, S. R., Anda, R. F., Felitti, V. J., Edwards, V. J., & Croft, J. B. (2002). Adverse childhood experiences and personal alcohol abuse as an adult. *Addictive Behaviors, 27*(5), 713–725. https://doi.org/10.1016/S0306-4603(01)00204-0

Duckworth, M. P., & Follette, V. M. (Eds.). (2011). *Retraumatization: Assessment, treatment, and prevention.* Routledge/Taylor & Francis Group. https://doi.org/10.4324/9780203866320

Due, C., Chiarolli, S., & Riggs, D. W. (2017). The impact of pregnancy loss on men's health and wellbeing: A systematic review. *BMC Pregnancy and Childbirth, 17*(1), 380. https://doi.org/10.1186/s12884-017-1560-9

Eadie, E. M., Runtz, M. G., & Spencer-Rodgers, J. (2008). Posttraumatic stress symptoms as a mediator between sexual assault and adverse health outcomes in undergraduate women. *Journal of Traumatic Stress, 21*(6), 540–547. https://doi.org/10.1002/jts.20369

Educational Testing Service. (n.d.). *Tele-assessment guidance for psychological, psychoeducational and neuropsychological assessment.* https://www.ets.org/pdfs/disabilities/tele-assessment-guidance.pdf

Edwards, V. J., Holden, G. W., Felitti, V. J., & Anda, R. F. (2003). Relationship between multiple forms of childhood maltreatment and adult mental health in community respondents: Results from the adverse childhood experiences study. *The American Journal of Psychiatry, 160*(8), 1453–1460. https://doi.org/10.1176/appi.ajp.160.8.1453

Eklund, K., Rossen, E., Koriakin, T., Chafouleas, S. M., & Resnick, C. (2018). A systematic review of trauma screening measures for children and adolescents. *School Psychology Quarterly, 33*(1), 30–43. https://doi.org/10.1037/spq0000244

El Baba, R., & Colucci, E. (2018). Post-traumatic stress disorders, depression, and anxiety in unaccompanied refugee minors exposed to war-related trauma: A systematic review. *International Journal of Culture and Mental Health, 11*(2), 194–207. https://doi.org/10.1080/17542863.2017.1355929

Elhai, J. D., Gold, S. N., Mateus, L. F., & Astaphan, T. A. (2001). Scale 8 elevations on the MMPI-2 among women survivors of childhood sexual abuse: Evaluating posttraumatic stress, depression, and dissociation as predictors. *Journal of Family Violence, 16*(1), 47–57. https://doi.org/10.1023/A:1026576425986

Elhai, J. D., Gold, S. N., Sellers, A. H., & Dorfman, W. I. (2001). The detection of malingered posttraumatic stress disorder with MMPI-2 fake bad indices. *Assessment, 8*(2), 221–236. https://doi.org/10.1177/107319110100800210

Elhai, J. D., Ruggiero, K. J., Frueh, B. C., Beckham, J. C., Gold, P. B., & Feldman, M. E. (2002). The Infrequency-Posttraumatic Stress Disorder scale (FPTSD) for the MMPI-2: Development and initial validation with veterans presenting with combat-related PTSD. *Journal of Personality Assessment, 79*(3), 531–549. https://doi.org/10.1207/S15327752JPA7903_08

Elklit, A., & Brink, O. (2004). Acute stress disorder as a predictor of post-traumatic stress disorder in physical assault victims. *Journal of Interpersonal Violence, 19*(6), 709–726. https://doi.org/10.1177/0886260504263872

Elliott, D. M. (1997). Traumatic events: Prevalence and delayed recall in the general population. *Journal of Consulting and Clinical Psychology, 65*(5), 811–820. https://doi.org/10.1037/0022-006X.65.5.811

Elliott, D. M., & Briere, J. (1994). Forensic sexual abuse evaluations of older children: Disclosures and symptomatology. *Behavioral Sciences & the Law, 12*(3), 261–277. https://doi.org/10.1002/bsl.2370120306

Elliott, D. M., & Briere, J. (1995). Posttraumatic stress associated with delayed recall of sexual abuse: A general population study. *Journal of Traumatic Stress, 8*(4), 629–647. https://doi.org/10.1002/jts.2490080407

Elliott, D. M., Mok, D. S., & Briere, J. (2004). Adult sexual assault: Prevalence, symptomatology, and sex differences in the general population. *Journal of Traumatic Stress, 17*(3), 203–211. https://doi.org/10.1023/B:JOTS.0000029263.11104.23

Engelhard, I. M., Arntz, A., & van den Hout, M. A. (2007). Low specificity of symptoms on the post-traumatic stress disorder (PTSD) symptom scale: A comparison of individuals with PTSD, individuals with other anxiety disorders and individuals without psychopathology. *British Journal of Clinical Psychology, 46*(Pt. 4), 449–456. https://doi.org/10.1348/014466507X206883

Ensink, K., Borelli, J. L., Normandin, L., Target, M., & Fonagy, P. (2020). Childhood sexual abuse and attachment insecurity: Associations with child psychological difficulties. *American Journal of Orthopsychiatry, 90*(1), 115–124. https://doi.org/10.1037/ort0000407

Epstein, M. A., & Bottoms, B. L. (2002). Explaining the forgetting and recovery of abuse and trauma memories: Possible mechanisms. *Child Maltreatment, 7*(3), 210–225. https://doi.org/10.1177/1077559502007003004

Epstein, R. S. (1993). Avoidant symptoms cloaking the diagnosis of PTSD in patients with severe accidental injury. *Journal of Traumatic Stress, 6*(4), 451–458. https://doi.org/10.1002/jts.2490060404

Epstein, R. S., Fullerton, C. S., & Ursano, R. J. (1998). Posttraumatic stress disorder following an air disaster: A prospective study. *The American Journal of Psychiatry, 155*(7), 934–938. https://doi.org/10.1176/ajp.155.7.934

Erwin, B. A., Heimberg, R. G., Juster, H., & Mindlin, M. (2002). Comorbid anxiety and mood disorders among persons with social anxiety disorder. *Behaviour Research and Therapy, 40*(1), 19–35. https://doi.org/10.1016/S0005-7967(00)00114-5

Exner, J. E. (2003). *The Rorschach: A comprehensive system: Vol. 1. Basic foundations and principles of interpretation* (4th ed.). Wiley.

Exner, J. E., Andronikof, A., & Fontan, P. (2022). *The Rorschach: A comprehensive system—Revised: Administration and coding manual.* Wiley.

Eytan, A., Guthmiller, A., Durieux-Paillard, S., Loutan, L., & Gex-Fabry, M. (2011). Mental and physical health of Kosovar Albanians in their place of origin: A post-war 6-year follow-up study. *Social Psychiatry and Psychiatric Epidemiology, 46*(10), 953–963. https://doi.org/10.1007/s00127-010-0269-0

Fairbank, J. A., Keane, T. M., & Malloy, P. F. (1983). Some preliminary data on the psychological characteristics of Vietnam veterans with posttraumatic stress disorders. *Journal of Consulting and Clinical Psychology, 51*(6), 912–919. https://doi.org/10.1037/0022-006X.51.6.912

Falsetti, S. A., & Resnick, H. S. (1997). Frequency and severity of panic attack symptoms in a treatment seeking sample of trauma victims. *Journal of Traumatic Stress, 10*(4), 683–689. https://doi.org/10.1002/jts.2490100414

Falsetti, S. A., Resnick, H. S., Kilpatrick, D. G., & Freedy, J. R. (1994). A review of the "Potential Stressful Events Interview": A comprehensive assessment instrument of high and low magnitude stressors. *Behavior Therapist, 17,* 66–67.

Farley, M. (2004a). Prostitution and trafficking in 9 countries: Update on violence and posttraumatic stress disorder. *Journal of Trauma Practice, 2,* 33–74.

Farley, M. (Ed.). (2004b). *Prostitution, trafficking, and traumatic stress.* Hayworth. https://doi.org/10.4324/9780203822463

Farley, M. (2017). Risks of prostitution: When the person is the product. *Journal of the Association for Consumer Research, 3*(1), 97–108.

Farley, M., & Barkan, H. (1998). Prostitution, violence, and posttraumatic stress disorder. *Women & Health, 27*(3), 37–49. https://doi.org/10.1300/J013v27n03_03

Farley, M., Cotton, A., Lynne, J., Zumbeck, S., Spiwak, F., Reyes, M. E., Alvarez, D., & Sezgin, U. (2004). Prostitution and trafficking in 9 countries: Update on violence and posttraumatic stress disorder. *Journal of Trauma Practice, 2*(3–4), 33–74. https://doi.org/10.1300/J189v02n03_03

Farren, J., Jalmbrant, M., Ameye, L., Joash, K., Mitchell-Jones, N., Tapp, S., Timmerman, D., & Bourne, T. (2016). Post-traumatic stress, anxiety and depression following miscarriage or ectopic pregnancy: A prospective cohort study. *BMJ Open, 6*(11), e011864. https://doi.org/10.1136/bmjopen-2016-011864

Felitti, V. J., & Anda, R. F. (2003). Relationship between multiple forms of childhood maltreatment and adult mental health in community respondents: Results from the Adverse Childhood Experiences study. *The American Journal of Psychiatry, 160*(8), 1453–1460. https://doi.org/10.1176/appi.ajp.160.8.1453

Felitti, V. J., Anda, R. F., Nordenberg, D., Williamson, D. F., Spitz, A. M., Edwards, V., Koss, M. P., & Marks, J. S. (1998). Relationship of childhood abuse and household dysfunction to many of the leading causes of death in adults: The Adverse Childhood Experiences (ACE) Study. *American Journal of Preventive Medicine, 14*(4), 245–258. https://doi.org/10.1016/S0749-3797 (98)00017-8

Fernandez, M. (2019, March 3). Braving heat and coyotes to be raped at the border. *The New York Times*, A1.

Filone, S., & DeMatteo, D. (2017). Assessing "credible fear": A psychometric examination of the Trauma Symptom Inventory-2 in the context of immigration court evaluations. *Psychological Assessment, 29*(6), 701–709.

Finkelhor, D., Shattuck, A., Turner, H. A., & Hamby, S. L. (2014). The lifetime prevalence of child sexual abuse and sexual assault assessed in late adolescence. *The Journal of Adolescent Health, 55*(3), 329–333. https://doi.org/10.1016/j.jadohealth.2013.12.026

Finzi-Dottan, R., & Karu, T. (2006). From emotional abuse in childhood to psychopathology in adulthood: A path mediated by immature defense mechanisms and self-esteem. *Journal of Nervous and Mental Disease, 194*(8), 616–621. https://doi.org/10.1097/01.nmd.0000230654.49933.23

Fiorentin, T. R., & Logan, B. K. (2019). Toxicological findings in 1000 cases of suspected drug facilitated sexual assault in the United States. *Journal of Forensic and Legal Medicine, 61*, 56–64. https://doi.org/10.1016/j.jflm.2018.11.006

First, M. B., Spitzer, R. L., Gibbon, M., & Williams, J. B. (1998). *Structured Clinical Interview for DSM-IV Axis I Disorders, Research Version, Patient Edition (SCID-I/P)*. Biometrics Research, New York State Psychiatric Institute.

First, M. B., Williams, J. B. W., Karg, R., & Spitzer, R. L. (2016). *Structured Clinical Interview for DSM-5 Disorders, Clinician Version (SCID-5-CV)*. American Psychiatric Association.

Fisher, P. M., Winne, P. H., & Ley, R. G. (1993). Group therapy for adult women survivors of child sexual abuse: Differentiation of completers versus dropouts. *Psychotherapy: Theory, Research, & Practice, 30*(4), 616–624. https://doi.org/10.1037/0033-3204.30.4.616

Fite, P. J., Stoppelbein, L., & Greening, L. (2009). Proactive and reactive aggression in a child psychiatric inpatient population. *Journal of Clinical Child and Adolescent Psychology, 38*(2), 199–205. https://doi.org/10.1080/15374410802698461

Fitzharris, M., Fildes, B., Charlton, J., & Tingvall, C. (2005). The relationship between perceived crash responsibility and post-crash depression. *Annual Proceedings of the Association for the Advancement of Automotive Medicine, 49*, 79–92.

Flory, J. D., & Yehuda, R. (2015). Comorbidity between post-traumatic stress disorder and major depressive disorder: Alternative explanations and treatment considerations. *Dialogues in Clinical Neuroscience, 17*(2), 141–150. https://doi.org/10.31887/DCNS.2015.17.2/jflory

Foa, E. B. (1995). *Posttraumatic Stress Diagnostic Scale*. National Computer Systems.

Foa, E. B., McLean, C. P., Zang, Y., Zhong, J., Powers, M. B., Kauffman, B. Y., Rauch, S., Porter, K., & Knowles, K. (2016a). Psychometric properties of the Posttraumatic Diagnostic Scale for *DSM-5* (PDS-5). *Psychological Assessment, 28*(10), 1166–1171. https://doi.org/10.1037/pas0000258

Foa, E. B., McLean, C. P., Zang, Y., Zhong, J., Rauch, S., Porter, K., Knowles, K., Powers, M. B., & Kauffman, B. Y. (2016b). Psychometric properties of the Posttraumatic Stress Disorder Symptom Scale Interview for *DSM-5* (PSSI-5). *Psychological Assessment, 28*(10), 1159–1165. https://doi.org/10.1037/pas0000259

Foa, E. B., & Tolin, D. F. (2000). Comparison of the PTSD Symptom Scale-Interview Version and the Clinician-Administered PTSD scale. *Journal of Traumatic Stress, 13*(2), 181–191. https://doi.org/10.1023/A:1007781909213

Follette, V. M., Polusny, M. A., Bechtle, A. E., & Naugle, A. E. (1996). Cumulative trauma: The impact of child sexual abuse, adult sexual assault, and spouse abuse. *Journal of Traumatic Stress, 9*(1), 25–35. https://doi.org/10.1002/jts.2490090104

Forbes, D., Creamer, M., & McHugh, T. (1999). MMPI-2 data for Australian Vietnam veterans with combat-related PTSD. *Journal of Traumatic Stress, 12*(2), 371–378. https://doi.org/10.1023/A:1024740929231

Ford, J. D. (2021). Polyvictimization and developmental trauma in childhood. *European Journal of Psychotraumatology, 12*(Suppl. 1), 1866394. https://doi.org/10.1080/20008198.2020.1866394

Ford, J. D., & Courtois, C. A. (Eds.). (2020). *Treating complex traumatic stress disorders in adults: Scientific foundations and therapeutic models* (2nd ed.). Guilford Press.

Ford, J. D., & Courtois, C. A. (2021). Complex PTSD and borderline personality disorder. *Borderline Personality Disorder and Emotion Dysregulation, 8*(1), 16. https://doi.org/10.1186/s40479-021-00155-9

Ford, J. D., Grasso, D. J., Elhai, J. D., & Courtois, C. A. (Eds.). (2015). Social, cultural, and other diversity issues in the traumatic stress field. In *Posttraumatic stress disorder: Scientific and professional dimensions* (2nd ed.). Academic Press. https://doi.org/10.1016/C2013-0-19408-1

Ford, J. D., & Hawke, J. (2015). Posttraumatic stress disorder and substance use disorders. In Y. Kaminer (Ed.), *Youth substance abuse and co-occurring disorders* (pp. 197–226). American Psychiatric Press.

Ford, J. D., & Kidd, P. (1998). Early childhood trauma and disorders of extreme stress as predictors of treatment outcome with chronic posttraumatic stress disorder. *Journal of Traumatic Stress, 11*(4), 743–761. https://doi.org/10.1023/A:1024497400891

Forke, C. M., Catallozzi, M., Localio, A. R., Grisso, J. A., Wiebe, D. J., & Fein, J. A. (2019). Intergenerational effects of witnessing domestic violence: Health of the witnesses and their children. *Preventive Medicine Reports, 15*, 100942. https://doi.org/10.1016/j.pmedr.2019.100942

Fowler, P. J., Tompsett, C. J., Braciszewski, J. M., Jacques-Tiura, A. J., & Baltes, B. B. (2009). Community violence: A meta-analysis on the effect of exposure and mental health outcomes of children and adolescents. *Development and Psychopathology, 21*(1), 227–259. https://doi.org/10.1017/S0954579409000145

Foy, D. W., Resnick, H. S., Sipprelle, R. C., & Carroll, E. M. (1987). Premilitary, military, and postmilitary factors in the development of combat-related posttraumatic stress disorder. *Behavior Therapist, 10*, 3–9.

Franklin, C. L., Repasky, S. A., Thompson, K. E., Shelton, S. A., & Uddo, M. (2002). Differentiating overreporting and extreme distress: MMPI-2 use with compensation-seeking veterans with PTSD. *Journal of Personality Assessment, 79*(2), 274–285. https://doi.org/10.1207/S15327752JPA7902_10

Friedrich, W. N. (2002). *Psychological assessment of sexually abused children and their families.* Sage. https://doi.org/10.4135/9781452233192

Frueh, B. C., Hamner, M. B., Cahill, S. P., Gold, P. B., & Hamlin, K. L. (2000). Apparent symptom overreporting in combat veterans evaluated for PTSD. *Clinical Psychology Review, 20*(7), 853–885. https://doi.org/10.1016/S0272-7358(99)00015-X

Fung, H. W., Yuan, G. F., Liu, C., Lin, E. S. S., Lam, S. K. K., & Wong, J. Y.-H. (2024). Prevalence and clinical correlates of dissociative symptoms in people with complex PTSD: Is complex PTSD a dissociative disorder? *Psychiatry Research, 339*, 116076. https://doi.org/10.1016/j.psychres.2024.116076

Gahm, G. A., Lucenko, B. A., Retzlaff, P., & Fukuda, S. (2007). Relative impact of adverse events and screened symptoms of posttraumatic stress disorder and depression among active duty soldiers seeking mental health care. *Journal of Clinical Psychology, 63*(3), 199–211. https://doi.org/10.1002/jclp.20330

Garcia, H. A., Franklin, C. L., & Chambliss, J. (2010). Examining MMPI-2 F-family scales in PTSD-diagnosed veterans of Operation Enduring Freedom and Operation Iraqi Freedom. *Psychological Trauma: Theory, Research, Practice, and Policy, 2*(2), 126–129. https://doi.org/10.1037/a0019155

Garvin, L. A., Greenan, M. A., Edelman, E. J., Slightam, C., McInnes, D. K., & Zulman, D. M. (2022). Increasing use of video telehealth among veterans experiencing homelessness with substance use disorder: Design of a peer-led intervention. *Journal of Technology in Behavioral Science, 8*(3), 234–245. https://doi.org/10.1007/s41347-022-00290-2

Gasquoine, P. G. (2009). Race-norming of neuropsychological tests. *Neuropsychology Review, 19*(2), 250–262. https://doi.org/10.1007/s11065-009-9090-5

Gauntlett-Gilbert, J., Keegan, A., & Petrak, J. (2004). Drug facilitated sexual assault: Cognitive approaches to treating the trauma. *Behavioural and Cognitive Psychotherapy, 32*(2), 215–223. https://doi.org/10.1017/S1352465804001481

Gilboa, D., Friedman, M., & Tsur, H. (1994). The burn as a continuous traumatic stress: Implications for emotional treatment during hospitalization. *Journal of Burn Care and Rehabilitation, 15*(1), 86–94. https://doi.org/10.1097/00004630-199401000-00017

Godbout, N., Daspe, M.-E., Runtz, M., Cyr, G., & Briere, J. (2019). Childhood maltreatment, attachment, and borderline personality-related symptoms: Gender-specific structural equation models. *Psychological Trauma: Theory, Research, Practice, and Policy, 11*(1), 90–98. https://doi.org/10.1037/tra0000403

Godbout, N., Hodges, M., Briere, J., & Runtz, M. (2016). Structural analysis of the Trauma Symptom Inventory–2. *Journal of Aggression, Maltreatment & Trauma, 25*(3), 333–346. https://doi.org/10.1080/10926771.2015.1079285

Godbout, N., Vaillancourt-Morel, M. P., Bigras, N., Briere, J., Hébert, M., Runtz, M., & Sabourin, S. (2019). Intimate partner violence in male survivors of child maltreatment: A meta-analysis. *Trauma, Violence & Abuse, 20*(1), 99–113. https://doi.org/10.1177/1524838017692382

Gold, S. N., Lucenko, B. A., Elhai, J. D., Swingle, J. M., & Sellers, A. H. (1999). A comparison of psychological/psychiatric symptomatology of women and men sexually abused as children. *Child Abuse & Neglect, 23*(7), 683–692. https://doi.org/10.1016/S0145-2134(99)00041-1

Goldstein, R. B., Smith, S. M., Chou, S. P., Saha, T. D., Jung, J., Zhang, H., Pickering, R. P., Ruan, W. J., Huang, B., & Grant, B. F. (2016). The epidemiology of DSM-5 posttraumatic stress disorder in the United States: Results from the National Epidemiologic Survey on Alcohol and Related Conditions-III. *Social Psychiatry and Psychiatric Epidemiology, 51*(8), 1137–1148. https://doi.org/10.1007/s00127-016-1208-5

Goodman, G. S., Ghetti, S., Quas, J. A., Edelstein, R. S., Alexander, K. W., Redlich, A. D., Cordon, I. M., & Jones, D. P. H. (2003). A prospective study of memory for child sexual abuse: New findings relevant to the repressed-memory controversy. *Psychological Science, 14*(2), 113–118. https://doi.org/10.1111/1467-9280.01428

Goodman, L. A., Corcoran, C., Turner, K., Yuan, N., & Green, B. L. (1998). Assessing traumatic event exposure: General issues and preliminary findings for the Stressful Life Events Screening Questionnaire. *Journal of Traumatic Stress, 11*(3), 521–542. https://doi.org/10.1023/A:1024456713321

Goodman, L. A., Saxe, L., & Harvey, M. (1991). Homelessness as psychological trauma: Broadening perspectives. *American Psychologist, 46*(11), 1219–1225. https://doi.org/10.1037/0003-066X.46.11.1219

Goodwin, B. E., Sellbom, M., & Arbisi, P. (2013). A posttraumatic stress disorder in veterans: The utility of the MMPI-2-RF validity scales in detecting over-reported symptoms. *Psychological Assessment, 25*(3), 671–678. https://doi.org/10.1037/a0032214

Gray, M., Litz, B., Hsu, J., & Lombardo, T. (2004). Psychometric properties of the Life Events Checklist. *Assessment, 11*(4), 330–341. https://doi.org/10.1177/1073191104269954

Green, B. L., Chung, J. Y., Daroowalla, A., Kaltman, S., & Debenedictis, C. (2006). Evaluating the cultural validity of the stressful life events screening questionnaire. *Violence Against Women, 12*(12), 1191–1213. https://doi.org/10.1177/1077801206294534

Green, B. L., Krupnick, J. L., Stockton, P., Goodman, L., Corcoran, C., & Petty, R. (2001). Psychological outcomes associated with traumatic loss in a sample of young women. *American Behavioral Scientist, 44*(5), 817–837. https://doi.org/10.1177/00027640121956511

Green, B. L., Lindy, J. D., Grace, M. C., Gleser, G. C., Leonard, A. C., Korol, M., & Winget, C. (1990). Buffalo Creek survivors in the second decade: Stability of stress symptoms. *American Journal of Orthopsychiatry, 60*(1), 43–54. https://doi.org/10.1037/h0079168

Green, B. L., & Solomon, S. D. (1995). The mental health impact of natural and technological disasters. In J. R. Freedy & S. E. Hobfoll (Eds.), *Traumatic stress: From theory to practice* (pp. 163–180). Plenum Press. https://doi.org/10.1007/978-1-4899-1076-9_7

Gregory, E. C. W., Valenzuela, C. P., & Hoyert, D. L. (2023). Fetal mortality: United States, 2021. *National Vital Statistics Report, 72*(8), 1–20.

Gros, D. F., Simms, L. J., & Acierno, R. (2010). Specificity of posttraumatic stress disorder symptoms: An investigation of comorbidity between posttraumatic stress disorder symptoms and depression in treatment-seeking veterans. *Journal of Nervous and Mental Disease, 198*(12), 885–890. https://doi.org/10.1097/NMD.0b013e3181fe7410

Groth-Marnat, G. (2003). *Handbook of psychological assessment* (4th ed.). John Wiley & Sons.

Grove, W. M., & Vrieze, S. I. (2009). An exploration of the base rate scores of the Millon Clinical Multiaxial Inventory-III. *Psychological Assessment, 21*(1), 57–67. https://doi.org/10.1037/a0014471

Guetta, R. E., Wilcox, E. S., Stoop, T. B., Maniates, H., Ryabchenko, K. A., Miller, M. W., & Wolf, E. J. (2019). Psychometric properties of the Dissociative Subtype of PTSD scale: Replication and extension in a clinical sample of trauma-exposed veterans. *Behavior Therapy, 50*(5), 952–966. https://doi.org/10.1016/j.beth.2019.02.003

Haahr-Pedersen, I., Perera, C., Hyland, P., Vallières, F., Murphy, D., Hansen, M., Spitz, P., Hansen, P., & Cloitre, M. (2020). Females have more complex patterns of childhood adversity: Implications for mental, social, and emotional outcomes in adulthood. *European Journal of Psychotraumatology, 11*(1), 1708618. https://doi.org/10.1080/20008198.2019.1708618

Hailes, H. P., Yu, R., Danese, A., & Fazel, S. (2019). Long-term outcomes of childhood sexual abuse: An umbrella review. *The Lancet Psychiatry, 6*(10), 830–839. https://doi.org/10.1016/S2215-0366(19)30286-X

Hall, H. (2024). Dissociation and misdiagnosis of schizophrenia in populations experiencing chronic discrimination and social defeat. *Journal of Trauma & Dissociation, 25*(3), 334–348. https://doi.org/10.1080/15299732.2022.2120154

Hall, J. E., Karch, D. L., & Crosby, A. E. (2016). *Elder abuse surveillance: Uniform definitions and recommended core data elements for use in elder abuse surveillance, Version 1.0.* National Center for Injury Prevention and Control, Centers for Disease Control and Prevention.

Hannah-Jones, N. (2021). *The 1619 Project: A new origin story.* One World.

Hanson, R. F., Kilpatrick, D. G., Falsetti, S. A., & Resnick, H. S. (1995). Violent crime and mental health. In J. R. Freedy & S. E. Hobfoll (Eds.), *Traumatic stress: From theory to practice* (pp. 129–161). Plenum Press. https://doi.org/10.1007/978-1-4899-1076-9_6

Hardesty, L., & Greif, G. L. (1994). Common themes in a group for female IV drug users who are HIV positive. *Journal of Psychoactive Drugs, 26*(3), 289–293. https://doi.org/10.1080/02791072.1994.10472443

Hardy, K. V., & Mueser, K. T. (2017). Trauma, psychosis and posttraumatic stress disorder. *Frontiers in Psychiatry, 8,* 220. https://doi.org/10.3389/fpsyt.2017.00220

Harrell, E. (2012). *Violent victimization committed by strangers, 1993–2010.* U.S. Department of Justice.

Hart, S. N., Brassard, M., Davidson, H. A., Rivelis, E., Diaz, V., & Binggeli, N. J. (2011). Psychological maltreatment. In J. E. B. Myers (Ed.), *American Professional Society on the Abuse of Children (APSAC) handbook on child maltreatment* (3rd ed., pp. 125–144). Sage.

Hartman, W. L., Clark, M. E., Morgan, M. K., Dunn, V. K., Fine, A. D., Perry, G. G., Jr., & Winsch, D. L. (1990). Rorschach structure of a hospitalized sample of Vietnam veterans with PTSD. *Journal of Personality Assessment, 54*(1–2), 149–159. https://doi.org/10.1207/s15327752jpa5401&2_15

Hartmann, W. E., Wendt, D. C., Burrage, R. L., Pomerville, A., & Gone, J. P. (2019). American Indian historical trauma: Anticolonial prescriptions for healing, resilience, and survivance. *American Psychologist, 74*(1), 6–19. https://doi.org/10.1037/amp0000326

Harvey, A. G., & Bryant, R. A. (1998). The relationship between acute stress disorder and posttraumatic stress disorder: A prospective evaluation of motor vehicle accident survivors. *Journal of Consulting and Clinical Psychology, 66*(3), 507–512. https://doi.org/10.1037/0022-006X.66.3.507

Harvey, A. G., & Bryant, R. A. (1999). Acute stress disorder across trauma populations. *Journal of Nervous and Mental Disease, 187*(7), 443–446. https://doi.org/10.1097/00005053-199907000-00009

Harvey, A. G., & Bryant, R. A. (2002). Acute stress disorder: A synthesis and critique. *Psychological Bulletin, 128*(6), 886–902. https://doi.org/10.1037/0033-2909.128.6.886

Hathaway, S. R., & McKinley, J. C. (1943). *The Minnesota Multiphasic Personality Inventory* (Rev. ed.). University of Minnesota Press.

Hauch, D., & Elklit, A. (2023, June 14). *The psychological consequences of stalking: Cross-sectional findings in a sample of Danish help-seeking stalking victims* [Poster presentation]. 17th European Society for Traumatic Stress Studies Conference, Belfast, Northern Ireland.

Haviland, M. G., Sonne, J. L., & Woods, L. R. (1995). Beyond posttraumatic stress disorder: Object relations and reality testing disturbances in physically and sexually abused adolescents. *Journal of the American Academy of Child & Adolescent Psychiatry, 34*(8), 1054–1059. https://doi.org/10.1097/00004583-199508000-00015

Hawes, S. W., & Boccaccini, M. T. (2009). Detection of overreporting of psychopathology on the Personality Assessment Inventory: A meta-analytic review. *Psychological Assessment, 21*(1), 112–124. https://doi.org/10.1037/a0015036

Hedtke, K. A., Ruggiero, K. J., Fitzgerald, M. M., Zinzow, H. M., Saunders, B. E., Resnick, H. S., & Kilpatrick, D. G. (2008). A longitudinal investigation of interpersonal violence in relation to mental health and substance use. *Journal of Consulting and Clinical Psychology, 76*(4), 633–647. https://doi.org/10.1037/0022-006X.76.4.633

Henderson, J. L., & Moore, M. (1944). The psychoneuroses of war. *The New England Journal of Medicine, 230*(10), 273–278. https://doi.org/10.1056/NEJM194403092301001

Herek, G. M., Gillis, J. R., & Cogan, J. C. (1999). Psychological sequelae of hate-crime victimization among lesbian, gay, and bisexual adults. *Journal of Consulting and Clinical Psychology, 67*(6), 945–951. https://doi.org/10.1037/0022-006X.67.6.945

Herman, D., Weathers, F., Litz, B., Joaquim, S., & Keane, T. (1993, October). *The PK Scale of the MMPI-2: Reliability and validity of the embedded and standalone versions* [Paper presentation]. Annual Meeting of the International Society for Traumatic Stress Studies, San Antonio, TX, United States.

Herman, J. L. (1992a). Complex PTSD: A syndrome in survivors of prolonged and repeated trauma. *Journal of Traumatic Stress, 5*(3), 377–391. https://doi.org/10.1002/jts.2490050305

Herman, J. L. (1992b). *Trauma and recovery: The aftermath of violence—From domestic abuse to political terror.* Basic Books.

Higson-Smith, C. (2015). *Updating the estimate of refugees resettled in the United States who have suffered torture.* The Center for Victims of Torture.

Hildenbrand, A. K., Nicholls, E. G., Aggarwal, R., Brody-Bizar, E., & Daly, B. P. (2015). Symptom Checklist-90-Revised (SCL-90-R). In R. L. Cautin & S. O. Lilienfeld (Eds.), *The encyclopedia of clinical psychology* (pp. 1–5). Wiley. https://doi.org/10.1002/9781118625392.wbecp495

Hinton, D. E., Kredlow, M. A., Pich, V., Bui, E., & Hofmann, S. G. (2013). The relationship of PTSD to key somatic complaints and cultural syndromes among Cambodian refugees attending a psychiatric clinic: The Cambodian Somatic Symptom and Syndrome Inventory (CSSI). *Transcultural Psychiatry, 50*(3), 347–370. https://doi.org/10.1177/1363461513481187

Hobfoll, S. E. (1988). *The ecology of stress.* Hemisphere.

Holeva, V., & Tarrier, N. (2001). Personality and peritraumatic dissociation in the prediction of PTSD in victims of road traffic accidents. *Journal of Psychosomatic Research, 51*(5), 687–692. https://doi.org/10.1016/S0022-3999(01)00256-2

Holmes, G. E., Williams, C. L., & Haines, J. (2001). Motor vehicle accident trauma exposure: Personality profiles associated with posttraumatic diagnoses. *Anxiety, Stress, & Coping, 14*(3), 301–313. https://doi.org/10.1080/10615800108248359

Holt, S., Buckley, H., & Whelan, S. (2008). The impact of exposure to domestic violence on children and young people: A review of the literature. *Child Abuse & Neglect, 32*(8), 797–810. https://doi.org/10.1016/j.chiabu.2008.02.004

Horowitz, M. D., Wilner, N., & Alvarez, W. (1979). Impacts of Event Scale: A measure of subjective stress. *Psychosomatic Medicine, 41*, 209–218.

Hyer, L., Boyd, S., Stanger, E., Davis, H., & Walters, P. (1997). Validation of the MCMI-III PTSD scale among combat veterans. *Psychological Reports, 80*(3, Pt 1), 720–722. https://doi.org/10.2466/pr0.1997.80.3.720

Hyer, L., Fallon, J., Harrison, W. R., & Boudewyns, P. (1987). MMPI overreporting by Vietnam combat veterans. *Journal of Clinical Psychology, 43*, 79–83.

Hyer, L., Woods, M. G., Boudewyns, P. A., Harrison, W. R., & Tamkin, A. S. (1990). MCMI and 16-PF with Vietnam veterans: Profiles and concurrent validation of MCMI. *Journal of Personality Disorders, 4*(4), 391–401. https://doi.org/10.1521/pedi.1990.4.4.391

Hynan, D. (2004). Unsupported gender differences on some personality disorder scales of the Millon Clinical Multiaxial Inventory-III. *Professional Psychology: Research and Practice, 35*(1), 105–110. https://doi.org/10.1037/0735-7028.35.1.105

Iloson, C., Möller, A., Sundfeldt, K., & Bernhardsson, S. (2021). Symptoms within somatization after sexual abuse among women: A scoping review. *Acta Obstetricia et Gynecologica Scandinavica, 100*(4), 758–767. https://doi.org/10.1111/aogs.14084

Ingram, P. B., Mosier, N. J., Sharpnack, J. D., & Golden, B. (2021). Evaluating symptom endorsement typographies of trauma-exposed veterans on the Personality Assessment Inventory: A latent profile analysis. *Current Psychology, 40*(11), 5267–5277. https://doi.org/10.1007/s12144-019-00486-5

Institute of Medicine. (2010). *Gulf War and health: Vol. 8. Health effects of serving in the Gulf War.* http://www.iom.edu/Reports/2010/Gulf-War-and-Health-Volume-8-Health-Effects-of-Serving-in-the-Gulf-War.aspx

Institute of Medicine, & National Research Council. (2013). *Confronting commercial sexual exploitation and sex trafficking of minors in the United States.* National Academies Press. https://doi.org/10.17226/18358

International Society for the Study of Trauma and Dissociation. (2011). Guidelines for treating dissociative identity disorder in adults, third revision, *Journal of Trauma & Dissociation, 12*(2), 115–187.

Janssen, H. J., Cuisinier, M. C., de Graauw, K. P., & Hoogduin, K. A. (1997). A prospective study of risk factors predicting grief intensity following pregnancy loss. *Archives of General Psychiatry, 54*(1), 56–61. https://doi.org/10.1001/archpsyc.1997.01830130062013

Jeve, Y. B., & Davies, W. (2014). Evidence-based management of recurrent miscarriages. *Journal of Human Reproductive Sciences, 7*(3), 159–169. https://doi.org/10.4103/0974-1208.142475

Joint Task Force for the Development of Telepsychology Guidelines for Psychologists. (2013). Guidelines for the practice of telepsychology. *American Psychologist, 68*(9), 791–800. https://doi.org/10.1037/a0035001

Jones, S. R., & Fernyhough, C. (2007). A new look at the neural diathesis—stress model of schizophrenia: The primacy of social–evaluative and uncontrollable situations. *Schizophrenia Bulletin, 33*(5), 1171–1177. https://doi.org/10.1093/schbul/sbl058

Jordan, R. G., Nunley, T. V., & Cook, R. R. (1992). Symptom exaggeration in a PTSD inpatient population: Response set or claim for compensation. *Journal of Traumatic Stress, 5*(4), 633–642. https://doi.org/10.1002/jts.2490050412

Kamphuis, J. H., Kugeares, S. L., & Finn, S. E. (2000). Rorschach correlates of sexual abuse: Trauma content and aggression indexes. *Journal of Personality Assessment, 75*(2), 212–224. https://doi.org/10.1207/S15327752JPA7502_3

Kang, H., Dalager, N., Mahan, C., & Ishii, E. (2005). The role of sexual assault on the risk of PTSD among Gulf War veterans. *Annals of Epidemiology, 15*(3), 191–195. https://doi.org/10.1016/j.annepidem.2004.05.009

Karam, E. G., Friedman, M. J., Hill, E. D., Kessler, R. C., McLaughlin, K. A., Petukhova, M., Sampson, L., Shahly, V., Angermeyer, M. C., Bromet, E. J., de Girolamo, G., de Graaf, R., Demyttenaere, K., Ferry, F., Florescu, S. E., Haro, J. M., He, Y., Karam, A. N., Kawakami, N., . . . Koenen, K. C. (2014). Cumulative traumas and risk thresholds: 12-month PTSD in the World Mental Health (WMH) surveys. *Depression and Anxiety, 31*(2), 130–142. https://doi.org/10.1002/da.22169

Karatzias, T., Shevlin, M., Fyvie, C., Hyland, P., Efthymiadou, E., Wilson, D., Roberts, N., Bisson, J. I., Brewin, C. R., & Cloitre, M. (2017). Evidence of distinct profiles of posttraumatic stress disorder (PTSD) and complex post-traumatic stress disorder (CPTSD) based on the new ICD-11 Trauma Questionnaire (ICD-TQ). *Journal of Affective Disorders, 207*, 181–187. https://doi.org/10.1016/j.jad.2016.09.032

Karatzias, T., Shevlin, M., Hyland, P., Fyvie, C., Grandison, G., & Ben-Ezra, M. (2021). ICD-11 posttraumatic stress disorder, complex PTSD and adjustment disorder: The importance of stressors and traumatic life events. *Anxiety, Stress, & Coping, 34*(2), 1–12. https://doi.org/10.1080/10615806.2020.1803006

Kaser-Boyd, N. (1993). Post-traumatic stress disorder in children and adults: The legal relevance. *Western State University Law Review, 20*, 319–334.

Kate, M.-A., Jamieson, G., Dorahy, M. J., & Middleton, W. (2021). Measuring dissociative symptoms and experiences in an Australian college sample using a short version of the multidimensional inventory of dissociation. *Journal of Trauma & Dissociation, 22*(3), 265–287. https://doi.org/10.1080/15299732.2020.1792024

Kealy, D., Rice, S. M., Ogrodniczuk, J. S., & Spidel, A. (2018). Childhood trauma and somatic symptoms among psychiatric outpatients: Investigating the role of shame and guilt. *Psychiatry Research, 268*, 169–174. https://doi.org/10.1016/j.psychres.2018.06.072

Keane, T. M., Fairbank, J. A., Caddell, J. M., Zimering, R. T., Taylor, K. L., & Mora, C. A. (1989). Clinical evaluation of a measure to assess combat exposure. *Psychological Assessment, 1*(1), 53–55. https://doi.org/10.1037/1040-3590.1.1.53

Keane, T. M., Malloy, P. F., & Fairbank, J. A. (1984). Empirical development of an MMPI subscale for the assessment of combat-related posttraumatic stress disorder. *Journal of Consulting and Clinical Psychology*, *52*(5), 888–891. https://doi.org/10.1037/0022-006X.52.5.888

Keen, M. A., Greene, T. E., Robinson, B. A., Morris, N. M., & Ingram, P. B. (2024). Assessment of PTSD and trauma symptoms with the MMPI-3: Validity and incremental utility of the Anxiety Related Experiences (ARX) scale. *Journal of Personality Assessment, 106(5)*, 561–573. https://doi.org/10.1080/00223891.2024.2315127

Kellner, M., & Yehuda, R. (1999). Do panic disorder and posttraumatic stress disorder share a common psychoneuroendocrinology? *Psychoneuroendocrinology*, *24*, 485–504.

Kendall, J. (2021, July 1). Forgotten memories of traumatic events get some backing from brain-imaging studies. *Scientific American*. https://www.scientificamerican.com/article/forgotten-memories-of-traumatic-events-get-some-backing-from-brain-imaging-studies/

Kendall-Tackett, K. (2009). Psychological trauma and physical health: A psychoneuroimmunology approach to etiology of negative health effects and possible interventions. *Psychological Trauma: Theory, Research, Practice, and Policy, 1*(1), 35–48. https://doi.org/10.1037/a0015128

Kendler, K. S., Myers, J., & Prescott, C. A. (2002). The etiology of phobias: An evaluation of the stress-diathesis model. *Archives of General Psychiatry*, *59*(3), 242–248. https://doi.org/10.1001/archpsyc.59.3.242

Keo-Meier, C. L., & Fitzgerald, K. M. (2017). Affirmative psychological testing and neurocognitive assessment with transgender adults. *The Psychiatric Clinics of North America*, *40*(1), 51–64. https://doi.org/10.1016/j.psc.2016.10.011

Keo-Meier, C. L., Herman, L. I., Reisner, S. L., Pardo, S. T., Sharp, C., & Babcock, J. C. (2015). Testosterone treatment and MMPI-2 improvement in transgender men: A prospective controlled study. *Journal of Consulting and Clinical Psychology*, *83*(1), 143–156. https://doi.org/10.1037/a0037599

Kessler, R. C., Sonnega, A., Bromet, E., Hughes, M., & Nelson, C. B. (1995). Posttraumatic stress disorder in the National Comorbidity Survey. *Archives of General Psychiatry*, *52*(12), 1048–1060. https://doi.org/10.1001/archpsyc.1995.03950240066012

Kilcommons, A. M., Morrison, A. P., Knight, A., & Lobban, F. (2008). Psychotic experiences in people who have been sexually assaulted. *Social Psychiatry and Psychiatric Epidemiology*, *43*(8), 602–611. https://doi.org/10.1007/s00127-007-0303-z

Kilpatrick, D. G., Resnick, H. S., Milanak, M. E., Miller, M. W., Keyes, K. M., & Friedman, M. J. (2013). National estimates of exposure to traumatic events and PTSD prevalence using *DSM-IV* and *DSM-5* criteria. *Journal of Traumatic Stress, 26*(5), 537–547. https://doi.org/10.1002/jts.21848

Kimerling, R., & Calhoun, K. S. (1994). Somatic symptoms, social support, and treatment seeking among sexual assault victims. *Journal of Consulting and*

Clinical Psychology, 62(2), 333–340. https://doi.org/10.1037/0022-006X. 62.2.333

King, C., Hill, S., Wolff, J., Bigony, C., Winternitz, S., Ressler, K., Kaufman, M., & Lebois, L. (2020). Childhood maltreatment type and severity predict depersonalization and derealization in treatment-seeking women with posttraumatic stress disorder. *Psychiatry Research, 292*, 113301. https://doi.org/10.1016/j.psychres.2020.113301

Kirmayer, L. J. (1996). Confusion of the senses: Implications of ethnocultural variation in somatoform and dissociative disorders for PTSD. In A. J. Marsella, M. J. Friedman, E. T. Gerrity, & R. M. Scurfield (Eds.), *Ethnocultural aspects of posttraumatic stress disorder: Issues, research, and clinical applications* (pp. 91–122). American Psychological Association. https://doi.org/10.1037/10555-005

Kirmayer, L. J., Kienzler, H., Afana, A. H., & Pedersen, D. (2010). Trauma and disasters in social and cultural context. In C. Morgan & D. Bhugra (Eds.), *Principles of Social Psychiatry* (pp. 155–177). Wiley Blackwell. https://doi.org/10.1002/9780470684214.ch13

Kisiel, C., Fehrenbach, T., Conradi, L., & Weil, L. (2021). *Trauma-informed assessment with children and adolescents: Strategies to support clinicians*. American Psychological Association. https://doi.org/10.1037/0000233-000

Kleijn, W. C., Hovens, J. E., & Rodenburg, J. J. (2001). Posttraumatic stress symptoms in refugees: Assessments with the Harvard Trauma Questionnaire and the Hopkins Symptom Checklist-25 in different languages. *Psychological Reports, 88*, 527–532.

Klest, B. (2012). Childhood trauma, poverty, and adult victimization. *Psychological Trauma: Theory, Research, Practice, and Policy, 4*(3), 245–251. https://doi.org/10.1037/a0024468

Klonoff, E. A., & Landrine, H. (1995). The Schedule of Sexist Events: A measure of lifetime and recent sexist discrimination in women's lives. *Psychology of Women Quarterly, 19*(4), 439–472. https://doi.org/10.1111/j.1471-6402.1995.tb00086.x

Klonsky E. D. (2007). The functions of deliberate self-injury: A review of the evidence. *Clinical Psychology Review, 27*(2), 226–239. https://doi.org/10.1016/j.cpr.2006.08.002

Klotz Flitter, J. M., Elhai, J. D., & Gold, S. N. (2003). MMPI-2 F scale elevations in adult victims of child sexual abuse. *Journal of Traumatic Stress, 16*(3), 269–274.

Kluft, R. P. (1993). Multiple personality disorder. In D. Spiegel, R. P. Kluft, R. Loewenstein, J. C. Nemiah, F. W. Putnam, & M. Steinberg (Eds.), *Dissociative disorders: A clinical review* (pp. 17–44). Sidran Press.

Koenen, K. C., Harley, R., Lyons, M. J., Wolfe, J., Simpson, J. C., Goldberg, J., Eisen, S. A., & Tsuang, M. (2002). A twin registry study of familial and individual risk factors for trauma exposure and posttraumatic stress disorder. *Journal of Nervous and Mental Disease, 190*(4), 209–218. https://doi.org/10.1097/00005053-200204000-00001

Koenig, H. G., & Al Zaben, F. (2021). Moral injury: An increasingly recognized and widespread syndrome. *Journal of Religion and Health, 60*(5), 2989–3011. https://doi.org/10.1007/s10943-021-01328-0

Koenig, H. G., Youssef, N. A., Ames, D., Oliver, J. P., Teng, E. J., Haynes, K., Erickson, Z. D., Arnold, I., Currier, J. M., O'Garo, K., & Pearce, M. (2018). Moral injury and religiosity in US veterans with posttraumatic stress disorder symptoms. *Journal of Nervous and Mental Disease, 206*(5), 325–331. https://doi.org/10.1097/NMD.0000000000000798

Koopman, C., Classen, C., Cardeña, E., & Spiegel, D. (1995). When disaster strikes, acute stress disorder may follow. *Journal of Traumatic Stress, 8*(1), 29–46. https://doi.org/10.1002/jts.2490080103

Koopman, C., Classen, C., & Spiegel, D. (1996). Dissociative responses in the immediate aftermath of the Oakland/Berkeley firestorm. *Journal of Traumatic Stress, 9*(3), 521–540. https://doi.org/10.1002/jts.2490090309

Koretzky, M. B., & Peck, A. H. (1990). Validation and cross-validation of the PTSD subscale of the MMPI with civilian trauma victims. *Journal of Clinical Psychology, 46*(3), 296–300. https://doi.org/10.1002/1097-4679(199005)46:3<296::AID-JCLP2270460308>3.0.CO;2-A

Koss, M. P. (1983). The scope of rape: Implications for the clinical treatment of victims. *The Clinical Psychologist, 53*, 88–91.

Koss, M. P. (1993). Detecting the scope of rape: A review of prevalence research methods. *Journal of Interpersonal Violence, 8*(2), 198–222. https://doi.org/10.1177/088626093008002004

Koss, M. P., Abbey, A., Campbell, R., Cook, S., Norris, J., Testa, M., Ullman, S., West, C., & White, J. (2006). *The Sexual Experiences Short Form Victimization (SES-SFV)*. University of Arizona.

Krebs, C. P., Lindquist, C. H., Warner, T. D., Fisher, B. S., & Martin, S. L. (2009). College women's experiences with physically forced, alcohol- or other drug-enabled, and drug-facilitated sexual assault before and since entering college. *Journal of American College Health, 57*(6), 639–647. https://doi.org/10.3200/JACH.57.6.639-649

Kremyar, A. J., Ben-Porath, Y. S., Sellbom, M., & Gervais, R. O. (2023). Assessing posttraumatic stress disorder symptom clusters with the Minnesota Multiphasic Personality Inventory-3 in a forensic disability sample. *Journal of Clinical Psychology, 79*(12), 2798–2822. https://doi.org/10.1002/jclp.23581

Krieger, N., & Sidney, S. (1996). Racial discrimination and blood pressure: The CARDIA Study of young Black and White adults. *American Journal of Public Health, 86*(10), 1370–1378. https://doi.org/10.2105/ajph.86.10.1370

Krieger, N., Smith, K., Naishadham, D., Hartman, C., & Barbeau, E. M. (2005). Experiences of discrimination: Validity and reliability of a self-report measure for population health research on racism and health. *Social Science & Medicine, 61*(7), 1576–1596. https://doi.org/10.1016/j.socscimed.2005.03.006

Kubany, E. S., Haynes, S. N., Leisen, M. B., Owens, J. A., Kaplan, A. S., Watson, S. B., & Burns, K. (2000). Development and preliminary validation of a brief broad-spectrum measure of trauma exposure: The Traumatic Life Events Questionnaire. *Psychological Assessment, 12*(2), 210–224. https://doi.org/10.1037/1040-3590.12.2.210

Kulkarni, J. (2017). Complex PTSD—A better description for borderline personality disorder? *Australasian Psychiatry, 25*(4), 333–335. https://doi.org/10.1177/1039856217700284

Lacoursiere, R. B. (1993). Diverse motives for fictitious post-traumatic stress disorder. *Journal of Traumatic Stress, 6*(1), 141–149. https://doi.org/10.1002/jts.2490060112

LaFauci Schutt, J. M., & Marotta, S. A. (2011). Personal and environmental predictors of posttraumatic stress in emergency management professionals. *Psychological Trauma: Theory, Research, Practice, and Policy, 3*(1), 8–15. https://doi.org/10.1037/a0020588

Lambert, M. V., Sierra, M., Phillips, M. L., & David, A. S. (2002). The spectrum of organic depersonalization: A review plus four new cases. *The Journal of Neuropsychiatry and Clinical Neurosciences, 14*(2), 141–154. https://doi.org/10.1176/jnp.14.2.141

Laumann, E. O., Leitsch, S. A., & Waite, L. J. (2008). Elder mistreatment in the United States: Prevalence estimates from a nationally representative study. *The Journals of Gerontology: Series B: Psychological Sciences and Social Sciences, 63*(4), S248–S254. https://doi.org/10.1093/geronb/63.4.S248

Leavitt, F. (2001). The development of the Somatoform Dissociation Index (SDI): A screening measure of dissociation using MMPI-2 items. *Journal of Trauma & Dissociation, 2*(3), 67–80. https://doi.org/10.1300/J229v02n03_05

Lensvelt-Mulders, G., van der Hart, O., van Ochten, J. M., van Son, M. J. M., Steele, K., & Breeman, L. (2008). Relations among peritraumatic dissociation and posttraumatic stress: A meta-analysis. *Clinical Psychology Review, 28*(7), 1138–1151. https://doi.org/10.1016/j.cpr.2008.03.006

Levin, A. P., Kleinman, S. B., & Adler, J. S. (2014). DSM-5 and posttraumatic stress disorder. *The Journal of the American Academy of Psychiatry and the Law, 42*(2), 146–158.

Levy, K. N., Johnson, B. N., Clouthier, T. L., Scala, J. W., & Temes, C. M. (2015). An attachment theoretical framework for personality disorders. *Canadian Psychology, 56*(2), 197–207. https://doi.org/10.1037/cap0000025

Lewis, K. L., & Grenyer, B. F. (2009). Borderline personality or complex posttraumatic stress disorder? An update on the controversy. *Harvard Review of Psychiatry, 17*(5), 322–328. https://doi.org/10.3109/10673220903271848

Liem, M., & Kunst, M. (2013). Is there a recognizable post-incarceration syndrome among released "lifers"? *International Journal of Law and Psychiatry, 36*(3–4), 333–337. https://doi.org/10.1016/j.ijlp.2013.04.012

Lindsay, D. S., & Briere, J. (1997). The controversy regarding recovered memories of childhood sexual abuse: Pitfalls, bridges, and future directions. *Journal of Interpersonal Violence, 12*(5), 631–647. https://doi.org/10.1177/088626097012005002

Lipschitz, D. S., Kaplan, M. L., Sorkenn, J., Chorney, P., & Asnis, G. M. (1996). Childhood abuse, adult assault, and dissociation. *Comprehensive Psychiatry, 37*(4), 261–266. https://doi.org/10.1016/s0010-440x(96)90005-x

Lissek, S., & van Meurs, B. (2015). Learning models of PTSD: Theoretical accounts and psychobiological evidence. *International Journal of Psychophysiology, 98*(3, Pt 2), 594–605. https://doi.org/10.1016/j.ijpsycho.2014.11.006

Litz, B. T., Contractor, A. A., Rhodes, C., Dondanville, K. A., Jordan, A. H., Resick, P. A., Foa, E. B., Young-McCaughan, S., Mintz, J., Yarvis, J. S., Peterson, A. L., & the STRONG STAR Consortium. (2018). Distinct trauma types in military service members seeking treatment for posttraumatic stress disorder. *Journal of Traumatic Stress, 31*(2), 286–295. https://doi.org/10.1002/jts.22276

Litz, B. T., Penk, W. E., Gerardi, R. J., & Keane, T. M. (1992). Assessment of posttraumatic stress disorder. In P. A. Saigh (Ed.), *Posttraumatic stress disorder: A behavioral approach to assessment and treatment* (pp. 54–80). Allyn & Bacon.

Litz, B. T., Penk, W. E., Walsh, S., Hyer, L., Blake, D. D., Marx, B., Keane, T. M., & Bitman, D. (1991). Similarities and differences between MMPI and MMPI-2 applications to the assessment of posttraumatic stress disorder. *Journal of Personality Assessment, 57*(2), 238–253. https://doi.org/10.1207/s15327752jpa5702_4

Litz, B. T., Stein, N., Delaney, E., Lebowitz, L., Nash, W. P., Silva, C., & Maguen, S. (2009). Moral injury and moral repair in war veterans: A preliminary model and intervention strategy. *Clinical Psychology Review, 29*(8), 695–706. https://doi.org/10.1016/j.cpr.2009.07.003

Loewenstein, R. J. (2018). Dissociation debates: Everything you know is wrong. *Dialogues in Clinical Neuroscience, 20*(3), 229–242. https://doi.org/10.31887/DCNS.2018.20.3/rloewenstein

Logan, T. K., Walker, R., Cole, J., & Leukefeld, C. (2002). Victimization and substance abuse among women: Contributing factors, interventions, and implications. *Review of General Psychology, 6*(4), 325–397. https://doi.org/10.1037/1089-2680.6.4.325

Longden, E., Branitsky, A., Moskowitz, A., Berry, K., Bucci, S., & Varese, F. (2020). The relationship between dissociation and symptoms of psychosis: A meta-analysis. *Schizophrenia Bulletin, 46*(5), 1104–1113. https://doi.org/10.1093/schbul/sbaa037

Loo, C. M., Fairbank, J. A., Scurfield, R. M., Ruch, L. O., King, D. W., Adams, L. J., & Chemtob, C. M. (2001). Measuring exposure to racism: Development and validation of a Race-Related Stressor Scale (RRSS) for Asian American Vietnam veterans. *Psychological Assessment, 13*(4), 503–520. https://doi.org/10.1037/1040-3590.13.4.503

Lötvall, R., Palmborg, Å., & Cardeña, E. (2022). A 20-years+ review of the Stanford Acute Stress Reaction Questionnaire (SASRQ): Psychometric properties and findings. *European Journal of Trauma & Dissociation, 6*(3), 100269. https://doi.org/10.1016/j.ejtd.2022.100269

Lucenko, B. A., Gold, S. N., & Cott, M. A. (2000). Relationship to perpetrator and posttraumatic symptomatology among sexual abuse survivors. *Journal of Family Violence, 15*(2), 169–179. https://doi.org/10.1023/A:1007542911767

Lui, P. P., & Quezada, L. (2019). Associations between microaggression and adjustment outcomes: A meta-analytic and narrative review. *Psychological Bulletin, 145*(1), 45–78. https://doi.org/10.1037/bul0000172

Luxenberg, T., & Levin, P. (2004). The role of the Rorschach in the assessment and treatment of trauma. In J. P. Wilson & T. M. Keane (Eds.), *Assessing psychological trauma and PTSD* (2nd ed., pp. 190–225). Guilford Press.

Luxton, D. D., Pruitt, L. D., & Osenbach, J. E. (2014). Best practices for remote psychological assessment via telehealth technologies. *Professional Psychology: Research and Practice, 45*(1), 27–35. https://doi.org/10.1037/a0034547

Lyons, J. A., & Keane, T. M. (1992). Keane PTSD scale: MMPI and MMPI-2 update. *Journal of Traumatic Stress, 5,* 111–117.

Maeda, M., & Higa, M. (2006). Transportation disasters and posttraumatic responses: A review of studies on major sea, air, and rail accidents. *Japanese Journal of Traumatic Stress, 4,* 49–60.

Maggiora Vergano, C., Lauriola, M., & Speranza, A. M. (2015). The Complex Trauma Questionnaire (ComplexTQ): Development and preliminary psychometric properties of an instrument for measuring early relational trauma. *Frontiers in Psychology, 6,* 1323. https://doi.org/10.3389/fpsyg.2015.01323

Mangiulli, I., Jelicic, M., Patihis, L., & Otgaar, H. (2021). Believing in dissociative amnesia relates to claiming it: A survey of people's experiences and beliefs about dissociative amnesia. *Memory, 29*(10), 1362–1374. https://doi.org/10.1080/09658211.2021.1987475

Mann, B. J. (1995). The North Carolina Dissociation Index: A measure of dissociation using items from the MMPI-2. *Journal of Personality Assessment, 64*(2), 349–359. https://doi.org/10.1207/s15327752jpa6402_13

March, J. S. (1993). What constitutes a stressor? The "criterion A" issue. In J. R. T. Davidson & E. B. Foa (Eds.), *Posttraumatic stress disorder: DSM-IV and beyond.* American Psychiatric Association.

Marmar, C. R., Weiss, D. S., & Metzler, T. (1997). The Peritraumatic Dissociative Experiences Questionnaire. In J. P. Wilson & T. M. Keane (Eds.), *Assessing psychological trauma and PTSD: A practitioner's handbook* (pp. 412–428). Guilford Press.

Marsella, A. J. (2010). Ethnocultural aspects of PTSD: An overview of concepts, issues, and treatments. *Traumatology, 16*(4), 17–26. https://doi.org/10.1177/1534765610388062

Marsella, A. J., Friedman, M. J., Gerrity, E. T., & Scurfield, R. M. (Eds.). (1996). *Ethnocultural aspects of posttraumatic stress disorder: Issues, research, and clinical applications.* American Psychological Association. https://doi.org/10.1037/10555-000

Marshall, G. N., & Schell, T. L. (2002). Reappraising the link between peritraumatic dissociation and PTSD symptom severity: Evidence from a longitudinal study of community violence survivors. *Journal of Abnormal Psychology, 111*(4), 626–636. https://doi.org/10.1037/0021-843X.111.4.626

Marshall, R. D., Schneier, F. R., Lin, S. H., Simpson, H. B., Vermes, D., & Liebowitz, M. (2000). Childhood trauma and dissociative symptoms in panic disorder. *The American Journal of Psychiatry, 157*(3), 451–453. https://doi.org/10.1176/appi.ajp.157.3.451

Martin, L., Byrnes, M., McGarry, S., Rea, S., & Wood, F. (2017). Social challenges of visible scarring after severe burn: A qualitative analysis. *Burns, 43*(1), 76–83. https://doi.org/10.1016/j.burns.2016.07.027

Martin, P. K., Schroeder, R. W., & Odland, A. P. (2015). Neuropsychologists' validity testing beliefs and practices: A survey of North American professionals. *The Clinical Neuropsychologist, 29*(6), 741–776. https://doi.org/10.1080/13854046.2015.1087597

McClanahan, S. F., McClelland, G. M., Abram, K. M., & Teplin, L. A. (1999). Pathways into prostitution among female jail detainees and their implications for mental health services. *Psychiatric Services, 50*(12), 1606–1613. https://doi.org/10.1176/ps.50.12.1606

McDevitt-Murphy, M. E., Weathers, F. W., Adkins, J. W., & Daniels, J. B. (2005). Use of the personality assessment inventory in assessment of posttraumatic stress disorder in women. *Journal of Psychopathology and Behavioral Assessment, 27*(2), 57–65. https://doi.org/10.1007/s10862-005-5380-2

McDevitt-Murphy, M. E., Weathers, F. W., Flood, A. M., Eakin, D. E., & Benson, T. A. (2007). The utility of the PAI and the MMPI-2 for discriminating PTSD, depression, and social phobia in trauma-exposed college students. *Assessment, 14*(2), 181–195. https://doi.org/10.1177/1073191106295914

McHugh, P. R. (2008). *Try to remember: Psychiatry's clash over meaning, memory, and mind.* Dana Press.

Mellman, T. A., David, D., Bustamante, V., Fins, A. I., & Esposito, K. (2001). Predictors of post-traumatic stress disorder following severe injury. *Depression and Anxiety, 14*(4), 226–231. https://doi.org/10.1002/da.1071

Meltzer-Brody, S., Churchill, E., & Davidson, J. R. T. (1999). Derivation of the SPAN, a brief diagnostic screening test for post-traumatic stress disorder. *Psychiatry Research, 88*(1), 63–70. https://doi.org/10.1016/S0165-1781(99)00070-0

Merriam-Webster. (n.d.). *Microaggression.* In Merriam-Webster.com dictionary. Retrieved May 24, 2023, from https://www.merriam-webster.com/dictionary/microaggression

Mertens, Y. L., & Daniels, J. K. (2022). The Clinician-Administered Dissociative States Scale (CADSS): Validation of the German version. *Journal of Trauma & Dissociation, 23*(4), 366–384. https://doi.org/10.1080/15299732.2021.1989111

Meyer, G. J., Viglione, D. J., Mihura, J. L, Erard, R. E., & Erdberg, P. (2011). *Rorschach Performance Assessment System: Administration, coding, interpretation, and technical manual.* Rorschach Performance Assessment System.

Meyers, J. E. B. (1996). Expert testimony. In J. Briere, L. Berliner, J. A. Bulkley, C. Jenny, & T. Reid (Eds.), *The APSAC handbook on child maltreatment* (pp. 319–340). Sage.

Miller, J., & Schwartz, M. D. (1995). Rape myths and violence against street prostitutes. *Deviant Behavior, 16*(1), 1–23. https://doi.org/10.1080/01639625.1995.9967984

Millon, T. (1983). *Millon Clinical Multiaxial Inventory manual.* Interpretive Scoring System.

Millon, T. (1987). *Manual for the MCMI-II* (2nd ed.). National Computer Systems.

Millon, T. (1994). *Manual for the MCMI-III* (3rd ed.). National Computer Systems.

Millon, T., Grossman, S., & Millon, C. (2015). *MCMI-IV: Millon Clinical Multiaxial Inventory manual.* Pearson Clinical Assessments.

Mohammadi, M. R., Hooshyari, Z., Delavar, A., Amanat, M., Mohammadi, A., Abasi, I., & Salehi, M. (2023). Diagnostic validity of Millon Clinical Multiaxial Inventory-IV (MCMI-IV). *Current Psychology, 42*(21), 18052–18060. https://doi.org/10.1007/s12144-022-02972-9

Mollica, R. F., Caspi-Yavin, Y., Bollini, P., Truong, T., Tor, S., & Lavelle, J. (1992). The Harvard Trauma Questionnaire: Validating a cross-cultural instrument for measuring torture, trauma, and posttraumatic stress disorder in Indochinese refugees. *Journal of Nervous and Mental Disease, 180*(2), 111–116. https://doi.org/10.1097/00005053-199202000-00008

Mollica, R. F., Caspi-Yavin, Y., Lavelle, J., Tor, S., Yang, T., Chan, S., Pham, T., Ryan, A., & de Marneffe, D. (1996). The Harvard Trauma Questionnaire (HTQ) manual: Cambodian, Laotian, and Vietnamese versions. *Torture, 6*(Suppl. 1), 19–33.

Monroe, J. (2005). Women in street prostitution: The result of poverty and the brunt of inequity. *Journal of Poverty, 9*(3), 69–88. https://doi.org/10.1300/J134v09n03_04

Mooney, M. (2017). Recognizing, treating, and preventing trauma in LGBTQ youth. *Journal of Family Strengths, 17*(2), 16. https://doi.org/10.58464/2168-670X.1363

Moore, B. A., & Penk, W. E. (Eds.). (2019). *Treating PTSD in military personnel: A clinical handbook* (2nd ed.). Guilford Press.

Moore, L. J., Sager, D., Keopraseuth, K., Chao, L. H., Riley, C., & Robinson, E. (2001). Rheumatological disorders and somatization in U.S. Mien and Lao refugees with depression and post-traumatic stress disorder: A cross-cultural comparison. *Transcultural Psychiatry, 38*(4), 481–505. https://doi.org/10.1177/136346150103800407

Moran, R., & Farley, M. (2018). Consent, coercion, and culpability: Is prostitution stigmatized work or an exploitive and violent practice rooted in sex, race, and class inequality? *Archives of Sexual Behavior, 48*(7), 1947–1953. https://doi.org/10.1007/s10508-018-1371-8

Morey, L. C. (1991). *Personality Assessment Inventory: Professional manual.* Psychological Assessment Resources.

Morey, L. C. (1996). *An interpretive guide to the Personality Assessment Inventory.* Psychological Assessment Resources.

Morey, L. C. (2007). *Personality Assessment Inventory: Professional manual* (2nd ed.). Psychological Assessment Resources.

Morgan, C., & Fisher, H. (2007). Environment and schizophrenia: Environmental factors in schizophrenia: Childhood trauma—A critical review. *Schizophrenia Bulletin, 33*(1), 3–10. https://doi.org/10.1093/schbul/sbl053

Morina, N., Akhtar, A., Barth, J., & Schnyder, U. (2018). Psychiatric disorders in refugees and internally displaced persons after forced displacement: A systematic review. *Frontiers in Psychiatry, 9*, 433. https://doi.org/10.3389/fpsyt.2018.00433

Mozley, S. L., Miller, M. W., Weathers, F. W., Beckham, J. C., & Feldman, M. E. (2005). Personality Assessment Inventory (PAI) profiles of male veterans with combat-related posttraumatic stress disorder. *Journal of Psychopathology and Behavioral Assessment, 27*(3), 179–189. https://doi.org/10.1007/s10862-005-0634-6

Munley, P. H., Bains, D. S., Bloem, W. D., & Busby, R. M. (1995). Post-traumatic stress disorder and the MMPI-2. *Journal of Traumatic Stress, 8*(1), 171–178.

Murphy, R. J. (2023). Depersonalization/derealization disorder and neural correlates of trauma-related pathology: A critical review. *Innovations in Clinical Neuroscience, 20*(1–3), 53–59.

Mychailyszyn, M. P., Brand, B. L., Webermann, A. R., Şar, V., & Draijer, N. (2021). Differentiating dissociative from non-dissociative disorders: A meta-analysis of the Structured Clinical Interview for DSM Dissociative Disorders (SCID-D). *Journal of Trauma & Dissociation, 22*(1), 19–34. https://doi.org/10.1080/15299732.2020.1760169

Myers, J. E. B. (2016). *Legal issues in clinical practice with victims of violence.* Guilford Press.

Nadal, K. L., & Mendoza, R. J. (2014). Internalized oppression and the lesbian, gay, bisexual, and transgender community. In E. J. R. David (Ed.), *Internalized oppression: The psychology of marginalized groups* (pp. 227–252). Springer.

Nader, K. O. (2004). Assessing traumatic experiences in children and adolescents: Self-reports of DSM PTSD criteria B–D symptoms. In J. P. Wilson & T. M. Keane (Eds.), *Assessing psychological trauma and PTSD* (2nd ed., pp. 513–537). Guilford Press.

Nagata, D. K., Kim, J. H. J., & Wu, K. (2019). The Japanese American wartime incarceration: Examining the scope of racial trauma. *American Psychologist, 74*(1), 36–48. https://doi.org/10.1037/amp0000303

Najarian, L. M., Goenjian, A. K., Pelcovitz, D., Mandel, F., & Najarian, B. (2001). The effect of relocation after a natural disaster. *Journal of Traumatic Stress, 14*(3), 511–526. https://doi.org/10.1023/A:1011108622795

Nakamura, N., Dispenza, F., Abreu, R., Ollen, E., Pantalone, D., Canillas, G., Gormley, B., & Vencill, J. (2022). The APA guidelines for psychological practice with sexual minority persons: An executive summary of the 2021 revision. *American Psychologist, 77*(8), 953–962. https://doi.org/10.1037/amp0000939

National Center for PTSD. (2024). *Trauma and stressor exposure measures.* https://www.ptsd.va.gov/professional/assessment/te-measures/index.asp

National Center on Elder Abuse. (2005). *Elder abuse prevalence and incidence.*

National Child Traumatic Stress Network. (2024). *All measure reviews.* https://www.nctsn.org/treatments-and-practices/screening-and-assessments/measure-reviews/all-measure-reviews

Nemeroff, C. B., Heim, C. M., Thase, M. E., Klein, D. N., Rush, A. J., Schatzberg, A. F., Ninan, P. T., McCullough, J. P., Jr., Weiss, P. M., Dunner, D. L., Rothbaum, B. O., Kornstein, S., Keitner, G., & Keller, M. B. (2003). Differential responses to psychotherapy versus pharmacotherapy in patients with chronic forms of major depression and childhood trauma. *Proceedings of the National Academy of Sciences of the United States of America, 100*(24), 14293–14296. https://doi.org/10.1073/pnas.2336126100

New, A. S., Triebwasser, J., & Charney, D. S. (2008). The case for shifting borderline personality disorder to Axis I. *Biological Psychiatry, 64*(8), 653–659. https://doi.org/10.1016/j.biopsych.2008.04.020

Nichter, M. (1981). Idioms of distress: Alternatives in the expression of psychosocial distress: Case study from South India. *Culture, Medicine and Psychiatry, 5*(4), 379–408. https://doi.org/10.1007/BF00054782

Nijenhuis, E. R. S., Spinhoven, P., Van Dyck, R., van der Hart, O., & Vanderlinden, J. (1996). The development and psychometric characteristics of the Somatoform Dissociation Questionnaire (SDQ-20). *Journal of Nervous and Mental Disease, 184,* 688–694.

Nijenhuis, E. R. S., Spinhoven, P., Van Dyck, R., van der Hart, O., & Vanderlinden, J. (1997). The development of the Somatoform Dissociation Questionnaire (SDQ-5) as a screening instrument for dissociative disorders. *Acta Psychiatrica Scandinavica, 96,* 311–318.

Nijenhuis, E. R. S., Spinhoven, P., Van Dyck, R., van der Hart, O., & Vanderlinden, J. (1998). Psychometric characteristics of the Somatoform Dissociation Questionnaire: A replication study. *Psychotherapy and Psychosomatics, 67,* 17–23.

Nilsson, D., Dahlström, Ö., Wadsby, M., & Bergh Johannesson, K. (2018). Evaluation of the Swedish Trauma Symptom Inventory-2 in a clinical and a student population. *European Journal of Trauma & Dissociation, 2*(2), 71–82. https://doi.org/10.1016/j.ejtd.2017.10.006

Norman, S. B., Griffin, B. J., Pietrzak, R. H., McLean, C., Hamblen, J. L., & Maguen, S. (2024). The Moral Injury and Distress Scale: Psychometric evaluation and initial validation in three high-risk populations. *Psychological Trauma: Theory, Research, Practice, and Policy, 16*(2), 280–291. https://doi.org/10.1037/tra0001533

Norrholm, S. D., Zalta, A., Zoellner, L., Powers, A., Tull, M. T., Reist, C., Schnurr, P. P., Weathers, F., & Friedman, M. J. (2021). Does COVID-19 count? Defining

Criterion A trauma for diagnosing PTSD during a global crisis. *Depression and Anxiety, 38*(9), 882–885. https://doi.org/10.1002/da.23209

Norris, F. H. (1992). Epidemiology of trauma: Frequency and impact of different potentially traumatic events on different demographic groups. *Journal of Consulting and Clinical Psychology, 60*(3), 409–418. https://doi.org/10.1037/0022-006X.60.3.409

Norris, F. H., & Hamblen, J. L. (2004). Standardized self-report measures of civilian trauma and PTSD. In J. P. Wilson & T. M. Keane (Eds.), *Assessing psychological trauma and PTSD* (pp. 63–102). Guilford Press.

Norris, F. H., & Thompson, M. P. (1995). Applying community psychology to the prevention of trauma and traumatic life events. In J. R. Freedy & S. E. Hobfoll (Eds.), *Traumatic stress: From theory to practice* (pp. 49–71). Plenum Press. https://doi.org/10.1007/978-1-4899-1076-9_3

Nunnally, J. C., & Bernstein, I. H. (1994). *Psychometric theory* (3rd ed.). McGraw Hill.

O'Donnell, M. L., Agathos, J. A., Metcalf, O., Gibson, K., & Lau, W. (2019). Adjustment disorder: Current developments and future directions. *International Journal of Environmental Research and Public Health, 16*(14), 2537. https://doi.org/10.3390/ijerph16142537

O'Donnell, M. L., Alkemade, N., Creamer, M., McFarlane, A. C., Silove, D., Bryant, R. A., Felmingham, K., Steel, Z., & Forbes, D. (2016). A longitudinal study of adjustment disorder after trauma exposure. *The American Journal of Psychiatry, 173*(12), 1231–1238. https://doi.org/10.1176/appi.ajp.2016.16010071

O'Donnell, M. L., Creamer, M., & Pattison, P. (2004). Posttraumatic stress disorder and depression following trauma: Understanding comorbidity. *The American Journal of Psychiatry, 161*(8), 1390–1396. https://doi.org/10.1176/appi.ajp.161.8.1390

Ogata, K., Ishikawa, T., Michiue, T., Nishi, Y., & Maeda, H. (2011). Posttraumatic symptoms in Japanese bereaved family members with special regard to suicide and homicide cases. *Death Studies, 35*(6), 525–535. https://doi.org/10.1080/07481187.2011.553327

Olff, M., Bakker, A., Frewen, P., Aakvaag, H., Ajdukovic, D., Brewer, D., Elmore Borbon, D. L., Cloitre, M., Hyland, P., Kassam-Adams, N., Knefel, M., Lanza, J. A., Lueger-Schuster, B., Nickerson, A., Oe, M., Pfaltz, M. C., Salgado, C., Seedat, S., & Wagner, A. (2020). Screening for consequences of trauma—An update on the Global Collaboration on Traumatic Stress. *European Journal of Psychotraumatology, 11*(1), 1752504. https://doi.org/10.1080/20008198.2020.1752504

Olio, K. A. (2004). The truth about "false memory syndrome." In P. J. Caplan & L. Cosgrove (Eds.), *Bias in psychiatric diagnosis* (pp. 163–169). Jason Aronson.

Open Society. (2019). *Understanding sex work in an open society.* https://www.opensocietyfoundations.org/explainers/understanding-sex-work-open-society

Ormerod, A. J., & Steel, J. (2018). Sexual assault in the military. In C. B Travis, J. W. White, A. Rutherford, W. S. Williams, S. L. Cook, & K. F. Wyche (Eds.),

APA handbook of the psychology of women: Perspectives on women's private and public lives (pp. 195–213). American Psychological Association https://doi.org/10.1037/0000060-011

Orr, S. P., Claiborn, J. M., Altman, B., Forgue, D. F., de Jong, J. B., Pitman, R. K., & Herz, L. R. (1990). Psychometric profile of posttraumatic stress disorder, anxious, and healthy Vietnam veterans: Correlations with psychophysiologic responses. *Journal of Consulting and Clinical Psychology, 58*(3), 329–335. https://doi.org/10.1037/0022-006X.58.3.329

Özdemir, B., Celik, C., & Oznur, T. (2015). Assessment of dissociation among combat-exposed soldiers with and without posttraumatic stress disorder. *European Journal of Psychotraumatology, 6*(1), 26657. https://doi.org/10.3402/ejpt.v6.26657

Ozer, E. J., Best, S. R., Lipsey, T. L., & Weiss, D. S. (2003). Predictors of post-traumatic stress disorder and symptoms in adults: A meta-analysis. *Psychological Bulletin, 129*(1), 52–73. https://doi.org/10.1037/0033-2909.129.1.52

Pad, R. A., Huprich, S. K., & Porcerelli, J. (2020). Convergent and discriminant validity of self-report and performance-based assessment of object relations. *Journal of Personality Assessment, 102*(6), 858–865. https://doi.org/10.1080/00223891.2019.1625909

Pai, A., Suris, A. M., & North, C. S. (2017). Posttraumatic stress disorder in the *DSM-5*: Controversy, change, and conceptual considerations. *Behavioral Sciences, 7*(1), 7. https://doi.org/10.3390/bs7010007

Paolucci, E. O., Genuis, M. L., & Violato, C. (2001). A meta-analysis of the published research on the effects of child sexual abuse. *The Journal of Psychology, 135*(1), 17–36. https://doi.org/10.1080/00223980109603677

Parlar, M., Frewen, P. A., Oremus, C., Lanius, R. A., & McKinnon, M. (2016). Dissociative symptoms are associated with reduced neuropsychological performance in patients with recurrent depression and a history of trauma exposure. *European Journal of Psychotraumatology 7*(1), 29061. https://doi.org/10.3402/ejpt.v7.29061

Pearlman, L. A. (2003). *Trauma and Attachment Belief Scale*. Western Psychological Services.

Pearlman, L. A., & Saakvitne, K. W. (1995). *Trauma and the therapist: Countertransference and vicarious traumatization in psychotherapy with incest survivors.* W. W. Norton & Company.

Pearson. (2021). *Telepractice and questionnaires or rating scales*. https://www.pearsonassessments.com/content/dam/school/global/clinical/us/assets/telepractice/guidance-documents/telepractice-and-questionnaires-or-rating-scales.pdf

Peirce, J. M., Burke, C. K., Stoller, K. B., Neufeld, K. J., & Brooner, R. K. (2009). Assessing traumatic event exposure: Comparing the Traumatic Life Events Questionnaire to the Structured Clinical Interview for *DSM-IV*. *Psychological Assessment, 21*(2), 210–218. https://doi.org/10.1037/a0015578

Pelcovitz, D., van der Kolk, B., Roth, S., Mandel, F., Kaplan, S., & Resick, P. (1997). Development of a criteria set and a Structured Interview for Disorders of

Extreme Stress (SIDES). *Journal of Traumatic Stress, 10*(1), 3–16. https://doi.org/10.1002/jts.2490100103

Pennebaker, J. W. (2018). Expressive writing in psychological science. *Perspectives on Psychological Science, 13*(2), 226–229. https://doi.org/10.1177/1745691617707315

Perrin, S., Van Hasselt, V. B., & Hersen, M. (1997). Validation of the Keane MMPI-PTSD Scale against DSM-III-R criteria in a sample of battered women. *Violence and Victims, 12*(1), 99–104. https://doi.org/10.1891/0886-6708.12.1.99

Petri, J. M., Weathers, F. W., Witte, T. K., & Silverstein, M. W. (2020). The Detailed Assessment of Posttraumatic Stress–Second Edition (DAPS-2): Initial psychometric evaluation in an MTurk-recruited, trauma-exposed community sample. *Assessment, 27*(6), 1116–1127. https://doi.org/10.1177/1073191119880963

Pezawas, L., Stamenkovic, M., Jagsch, R., Ackerl, S., Putz, C., Stelzer, B., Moffat, R. R., Schindler, S., Aschauer, H., & Kasper, S. (2002). A longitudinal view of triggers and thresholds of suicidal behavior in depression. *The Journal of Clinical Psychiatry, 63*(10), 866–873. https://doi.org/10.4088/JCP.v63n1003

Phillips, C. J., Leardmann, C. A., Gumbs, G. R., & Smith, B. (2010). Risk factors for posttraumatic stress disorder among deployed US male Marines. *BMC Psychiatry, 10*(1), 52. https://doi.org/10.1186/1471-244X-10-52

Phillips, D. W. (1994). Initial development and validation of the Phillips Dissociation Scale (PDS) of the MMPI. *Progress in the Dissociative Disorders, 7*(2), 92–100.

Pickens, J., Field, T., Prodromidis, M., Pelaez-Nogueras, M., & Hossain, Z. (1995). Posttraumatic stress, depression and social support among college students after Hurricane Andrew. *Journal of College Student Development, 36*(2), 152–161.

Pieterse, A. L., Roberson, K. L., Garcia, R., & Carter, R. T. (2023). Racial discrimination and trauma symptoms: Further support for the Race-Based Traumatic Stress Symptom Scale. *Cultural Diversity & Ethnic Minority Psychology, 29*(3), 332–338. https://doi.org/10.1037/cdp0000544

Popovic, D., Schmitt, A., Kaurani, L., Senner, F., Papiol, S., Malchow, B., Fischer, A., Schulze, T. G., Koutsouleris, N., & Falkai, P. (2019). Childhood trauma in schizophrenia: Current findings and research perspectives. *Frontiers in Neuroscience, 13*, 274. https://doi.org/10.3389/fnins.2019.00274

Prachason, T., Mutlu, I., Fusar-Poli, L., Menne-Lothmann, C., Decoster, J., van Winkel, R., Collip, D., Delespaul, P., De Hert, M., Derom, C., Thiery, E., Jacobs, N., Wichers, M., van Os, J., Rutten, B. P. F., Pries, L., & Guloksuz, S. (2024). Gender differences in the associations between childhood adversity and psychopathology in the general population. *Social Psychiatry and Psychiatric Epidemiology, 59*(5), 847–858. https://doi.org/10.1007/s00127-023-02546-5

Prigerson, H. G., Bierhals, A. J., Kasl, S. V., Reynolds, C. F., III, Shear, M. K., Day, N., Beery, L. C., Newsom, J. T., & Jacobs, S. (1997). Traumatic grief as a risk factor for mental and physical morbidity. *American Journal of Psychiatry, 154*(5), 616–623. https://doi.org/10.1176/ajp.154.5.616

Prigerson, H. G., Boelen, P. A., Xu, J., Smith, K. V., & Maciejewski, P. K. (2021). Validation of the new *DSM-5-TR* criteria for prolonged grief disorder and the PG-13-Revised (PG-13-R) scale. *World Psychiatry, 20*(1), 96–106. https://doi.org/10.1002/wps.20823

Prigerson, H. G., & Jacobs, S. C. (2001). Traumatic grief as a distinct disorder: A rationale, consensus criteria, and a preliminary empirical test. In M. S. Stroebe, R. O. Hansson, W. Stroebe, & H. A. W. Schut (Eds.), *Handbook of bereavement research: Consequences, coping, and care* (pp. 613–645). American Psychological Association.

Prigerson, H. G., Maciejewski, P. K., Reynolds, C. F., III, Bierhals, A. J., Newsom, J. T., Fasiczka, A., Frank, E., Doman, J., & Miller, M. (1995). Inventory of Complicated Grief: A scale to measure maladaptive symptoms of loss. *Psychiatry Research, 59*(1–2), 65–79. https://doi.org/10.1016/0165-1781(95)02757-2

Prigerson, H. G., Shear, M. K., Jacobs, S. C., Reynolds, C. F., III, Maciejewski, P. K., Davidson, J. R. T., Rosenheck, R., Pilkonis, P. A., Wortman, C. B., Williams, J. B. W., Widiger, T. A., Frank, E., Kupfer, D. J., & Zisook, S. (1999). Consensus criteria for traumatic grief: A preliminary empirical test. *The British Journal of Psychiatry, 174*(1), 67–73. https://doi.org/10.1192/bjp.174.1.67

Prins, A., Bovin, M. J., Kimerling, R., Kaloupek, D. G., Marx, B. P., Pless Kaiser, A., & Schnurr, P. P. (2015). *The Primary Care PTSD Screen for DSM-5 (PC-PTSD-5)*. National Center for PTSD.

The Protection Project. (2011). *The Protection Project review of the Trafficking in Persons Report*. Johns Hopkins University.

Putnam, F. W., Guroff, J. J., Silberman, E. K., Barban, L., & Post, R. M. (1986). The clinical phenomenology of multiple personality disorder: Review of 100 recent cases. *The Journal of Clinical Psychiatry, 47*(6), 285–293.

Qassem, T., Aly-ElGabry, D., Alzarouni, A., Abdel-Aziz, K., & Arnone, D. (2021). Psychiatric co-morbidities in post-traumatic stress disorder: Detailed findings from the Adult Psychiatric Morbidity Survey in the English population. *Psychiatric Quarterly, 92*(1), 321–330. https://doi.org/10.1007/s11126-020-09797-4

Rademaker, A., Kleber, R., Meijer, M., & Vermetten, E. (2009). Investigating the MMPI–2 Trauma Profile in treatment-seeking peacekeepers. *Journal of Personality Assessment, 91*, 593–600. https://doi.org/10.1080/00223890903230899

Rausch, K., & Knutson, J. F. (1991). The self-report of personal punitive childhood experiences and those of siblings. *Child Abuse & Neglect, 15*(1–2), 29–36. https://doi.org/10.1016/0145-2134(91)90087-T

Read, J., Perry, B. D., Moskowitz, A., & Connolly, J. (2001). The contribution of early traumatic events to schizophrenia in some patients: A traumagenic neurodevelopmental model. *Psychiatry, 64*(4), 319–345. https://doi.org/10.1521/psyc.64.4.319.18602

Rees, S., Silove, D., Chey, T., Ivancic, L., Steel, Z., Creamer, M., Teesson, M., Bryant, R., McFarlane, A. C., Mills, K. L., Slade, T., Carragher, N., O'Donnell, M., & Forbes, D. (2011). Lifetime prevalence of gender-based violence in women and the relationship with mental disorders and psychosocial function. *JAMA*, *306*(5), 513–521. https://doi.org/10.1001/jama.2011.1098

Resick, P. A., Bovin, M. J., Calloway, A. L., Dick, A. M., King, M. W., Mitchell, K. S., Suvak, M. K., Wells, S. Y., Stirman, S. W., & Wolf, E. J. (2012). A critical evaluation of the complex PTSD literature: Implications for *DSM-5*. *Journal of Traumatic Stress*, *25*(3), 241–251. https://doi.org/10.1002/jts.21699

Resnick, H. S., Best, C. L., Kilpatrick, D. G., Freedy, J. R., & Falsetti, S. A. (1996). Trauma assessment for adults. In B. Hudnall Stamm (Ed.), *Measurement of stress, trauma, and adaptation* (pp. 362–365). Sidran Press.

Resnick, H. S., Falsetti, S. A., Kilpatrick, D. G., & Freedy, J. R. (1996). Assessment of rape and other civilian trauma-related post-traumatic stress disorder: Emphasis on assessment of potentially traumatic events. In T. W. Miller (Ed.), *Stressful life events* (pp. 231–266). International Universities Press.

Resnick, H. S., Kilpatrick, D. G., Dansky, B. S., Saunders, B. E., & Best, C. L. (1993). Prevalence of civilian trauma and posttraumatic stress disorder in a representative national sample of women. *Journal of Consulting and Clinical Psychology*, *61*(6), 984–991. https://doi.org/10.1037/0022-006X.61.6.984

Riggs, D. S., Kilpatrick, D. G., & Resnick, H. S. (1992). Long-term psychological distress associated with marital rape and aggravated assault: A comparison to other crime victims. *Journal of Family Violence*, *7*(4), 283–296. https://doi.org/10.1007/BF00994619

Rix, R. (2000). *Sexual abuse litigation: A practical resource for attorneys, clinicians, and advocates*. Routledge.

Roberts, A. L., Gilman, S. E., Breslau, J., Breslau, N., & Koenen, K. C. (2011). Race/ethnic differences in exposure to traumatic events, development of post-traumatic stress disorder, and treatment-seeking for post-traumatic stress disorder in the United States. *Psychological Medicine*, *41*(1), 71–83. https://doi.org/10.1017/S0033291710000401

Robinson, J., & Rubin, L. (2016). Homonegative microaggressions and post-traumatic stress symptoms. *Journal of Gay & Lesbian Mental Health*, *20*(1), 57–69. https://doi.org/10.1080/19359705.2015.1066729

Rogers, R., Sewell, K. W., & Gillard, N. D. (2010). *Structured Interview of Reported Symptoms* (2nd ed.). Psychological Assessment Resources.

Rorschach, H. (1981). *Psychodiagnostics: A diagnostic test based upon perception* (P. Lemkau & B. Kronemberg, Eds. & Trans.; 9th ed.). Grune & Stratton. (Original work published 1921)

Rosenbaum, D. L., & White, K. S. (2013). The role of anxiety in binge eating behavior: A critical examination of theory and empirical literature. *Health Psychology Research*, *1*(2), e19. https://doi.org/10.4081/hpr.2013.e19

Ross, C. A. (n.d.). *Dissociative Disorders Interview Schedule, DSM-5 version*. https://www.rossinst.com/downloads/DDIS-DSM-5.pdf

Ross, C. A. (1997). *Dissociative identity disorder: Diagnosis, clinical features, and treatment of multiple personality* (2nd ed.). John Wiley & Sons.

Ross, C. A. (2021). The dissociative taxon and dissociative identity disorder. *Journal of Trauma & Dissociation, 22*(5), 555–562. https://doi.org/10.1080/15299732.2020.1869645

Ross, C. A., & Browning, L. (2016). The Self-Report Dissociative Disorders Interview Schedule: A preliminary report. *Journal of Trauma & Dissociation, 18*(1), 31–37. https://doi.org/10.1080/15299732.2016.1172538

Ross, C. A., Duffy, C. M. M., & Ellason, J. W. (2002). Prevalence, reliability and validity of dissociative disorders in an inpatient setting. *Journal of Trauma & Dissociation, 3*(1), 7–17. https://doi.org/10.1300/J229v03n01_02

Ross, C. A., Heber, S., Norton, G. R., Anderson, D., & Barchet, P. (1989). The Dissociative Disorders Interview Schedule: A structured interview. *Dissociation, 2,* 169–189.

Russell, D. N., & Morey, L. C. (2019). Use of validity indicators on the Personality Assessment Inventory to detect feigning of post-traumatic stress disorder. *Psychological Injury and Law, 12*(3–4), 204–211. https://doi.org/10.1007/s12207-019-09349-7

Russell, S. T., & Fish, J. N. (2016). Mental health in lesbian, gay, bisexual, and transgender (LGBT) youth. *Annual Review of Clinical Psychology, 12*(1), 465–487. https://doi.org/10.1146/annurev-clinpsy-021815-093153

Saggino, A., Molinengo, G., Rogier, G., Garofalo, C., Loera, B., Tommasi, M., & Velotti, P. (2020). Improving the psychometric properties of the dissociative experiences scale (DES-II): A Rasch validation study. *BMC Psychiatry, 20*(1), 8. https://doi.org/10.1186/s12888-019-2417-8

Sanders, S. (1986). The Perceptual Alteration Scale: A scale measuring dissociation. *The American Journal of Clinical Hypnosis, 29*(2), 95–102. https://doi.org/10.1080/00029157.1986.10402691

Santiago, P. N., Ursano, R. J., Gray, C. L., Pynoos, R. S., Spiegel, D., Lewis-Fernandez, R., Friedman, M. J., & Fullerton, C. S. (2013). A systematic review of PTSD prevalence and trajectories in *DSM-5* defined trauma exposed populations: Intentional and non-intentional traumatic events. *PLoS One, 8*(4), e59236. https://doi.org/10.1371/journal.pone.0059236

Santina, M. R. (1998). *Object relations, ego development, and affect regulation in severely addicted substance abusers* [Unpublished doctoral dissertation]. Department of Psychology, Columbia University.

Sargant, W., & Slater, E. (1941). Amnestic syndromes in war. *Proceedings of the Royal Society of Medicine, 34*(12), 757–764. https://doi.org/10.1177/003591574103401202

Saunders, B. E., Arata, C. M., & Kilpatrick, D. G. (1990). Development of a crime-related post-traumatic stress disorder scale for women within the Symptom Checklist-90-Revised. *Journal of Traumatic Stress, 3*(3), 267–277.

Saunders, E. A. (1991). Rorschach indicators of chronic childhood sexual abuse in female borderline inpatients. *Bulletin of the Menninger Clinic, 55*(1), 48–71.

Sawyer, I. (2009). Soldiers who rape, commanders who condone. *Human Rights Watch.* https://www.hrw.org/report/2009/07/16/soldiers-who-rape-commanders-who-condone/sexual-violence-and-military-reform

Schalinski, I., Elbert, T., & Schauer, M. (2011). Female dissociative responding to extreme sexual violence in a chronic crisis setting: The case of Eastern Congo. *Journal of Traumatic Stress, 24*(2), 235–238. https://doi.org/10.1002/jts. 20631

Scheer, J. R., Batchelder, A. W., Wang, K., & Pachankis, J. E. (2022). Mental health, alcohol use, and substance use correlates of sexism in a sample of gender-diverse sexual minority women. *Psychology of Sexual Orientation and Gender Diversity, 9*(2), 222–235. https://doi.org/10.1037/sgd0000477

Scheibe, S., Bagby, R. M., Miller, L. S., & Dorian, B. J. (2001). Assessing posttraumatic stress disorder with the MMPI-2 in a sample of workplace accident victims. *Psychological Assessment, 13*(3), 369–374. https://doi.org/10.1037/1040-3590.13.3.369

Scher, C. D., Stein, M. B., Asmundson, G. J., McCreary, D. R., & Forde, D. R. (2001). The childhood trauma questionnaire in a community sample: Psychometric properties and normative data. *Journal of Traumatic Stress, 14*(4), 843–857. https://doi.org/10.1023/A:1013058625719

Schlenger, W., & Kulka, R. A. (1989). *PTSD scale development for the MMPI-2.* Research Triangle Park Institute.

Scoboria, A., Ford, J., Lin, H. J., & Frisman, L. (2008). Exploratory and confirmatory factor analyses of the structured interview for disorders of extreme stress. *Assessment, 15*(4), 404–425. https://doi.org/10.1177/1073191108319005

Scotti, J. R., Sturges, L. V., & Lyons, J. A. (1996). The Keane PTSD Scale extracted from the MMPI: Sensitivity and specificity with Vietnam veterans. *Journal of Traumatic Stress, 9*(3), 643–650. https://doi.org/10.1002/jts. 2490090320

Shabani, A., Masoumian, S., Zamirinejad, S., Hejri, M., Pirmorad, T., & Yaghmaeezadeh, H. (2021). Psychometric properties of Structured Clinical Interview for DSM-5 Disorders-Clinician Version (SCID-5-CV). *Brain and Behavior, 11*(5), e01894. https://doi.org/10.1002/brb3.1894

Shalev, A. Y., Peri, T., Canetti, L., & Schreiber, S. (1996). Predictors of PTSD in injured trauma survivors: A prospective study. *The American Journal of Psychiatry, 153*(2), 219–225. https://doi.org/10.1176/ajp.153.2.219

Shay, J. (1995). *Achilles in Vietnam: Combat trauma and the undoing of character.* New Touchstone.

Shay, J. (2014). Moral injury. *Psychoanalytic Psychology, 31*(2), 182–191. https://doi.org/10.1037/a0036090

Shear, M. K., & Smith-Caroff, K. (2002). Traumatic loss and the syndrome of complicated grief. *PTSD Research Quarterly, 13*, 1–7.

Shedler, J., Mayman, M., & Manis, M. (1993). The illusion of mental health. *The American Psychologist, 48*(11), 1117–1131. https://doi.org/10.1037//0003-066x.48.11.1117

Shepard, M. F., & Campbell, J. A. (1992). The Abusive Behavior Inventory: A measure of psychological and physical abuse. *Journal of Interpersonal Violence, 7*(3), 291–305. https://doi.org/10.1177/088626092007003001

Shevlin, M., Hyland, P., Roberts, N. P., Bisson, J. I., Brewin, C. R., & Cloitre, M. (2018). A psychometric assessment of Disturbances in Self-Organization symptom indicators for ICD-11 complex PTSD using the International Trauma Questionnaire. *European Journal of Psychotraumatology, 9*(1), 1419749. https://doi.org/10.1080/20008198.2017.1419749

Shinn, A. K., Wolff, J. D., Hwang, M., Lebois, L. A. M., Robinson, M. A., Winternitz, S. R., Öngür, D., Ressler, K. J., & Kaufman, M. L. (2019). Assessing voice hearing in trauma spectrum disorders: A comparison of two measures and a review of the literature. *Frontiers in Psychiatry, 10*, 1011. https://doi.org/10.3389/fpsyt.2019.01011

Silove, D., Baker, J. R., Mohsin, M., Teesson, M., Creamer, M., O'Donnell, M., Forbes, D., Carragher, N., Slade, T., Mills, K., Bryant, R., McFarlane, A., Steel, Z., Felmingham, K., & Rees, S. (2017). The contribution of gender-based violence and network trauma to gender differences in post-traumatic stress disorder. *PLoS One, 12*(2), e0171879. https://doi.org/10.1371/journal.pone.0171879

Simeon, D., Guralnik, O., & Schmeidler, J. (2001). Development of a depersonalization severity scale. *Journal of Traumatic Stress, 14*(2), 341–349. https://doi.org/10.1023/A:1011169019614

Simon, N. M., Hoeppner, S. S., Lubin, R. E., Robinaugh, D. J., Malgaroli, M., Norman, S. B., Acierno, R., Goetter, E. M., Hellberg, S. N., Charney, M. E., Bui, E., Baker, A. W., Smith, E., Kim, H. M., & Rauch, S. A. M. (2020). Understanding the impact of complicated grief on combat related posttraumatic stress disorder, guilt, suicide, and functional impairment in a clinical trial of post-9/11 service members and veterans. *Depression and Anxiety, 37*(1), 63–72. https://doi.org/10.1002/da.22911

Simon, R. I. (Ed.). (2003). *Posttraumatic stress disorder in litigation: Guidelines for forensic assessment* (2nd ed.). American Psychiatric Publishing, Inc.

Simpson, J. A., & Rholes, W. S. (Eds.). (2015). *Attachment theory and research: New directions and emerging themes.* Guilford Press.

Simpson, T. L., Comtois, K. A., Moore, S. A., & Kaysen, D. (2011). Comparing the diagnosis of PTSD when assessing worst versus multiple traumatic events in a chronically mentally ill sample. *Journal of Traumatic Stress, 24*(3), 361–364. https://doi.org/10.1002/jts.20647

Sloan, D. M., & Marx, B. P. (2019). *Written exposure therapy for PTSD: A brief treatment approach for mental health professionals.* American Psychological Association. https://doi.org/10.1037/0000139-000

Smith, D. W., & Frueh, B. C. (1996). Compensation seeking, comorbidity, and apparent exaggeration of PTSD symptoms among Vietnam combat veterans. *Psychological Assessment, 8*(1), 3–6. https://doi.org/10.1037/1040-3590.8.1.3

Smith, S. G., Chen, J., Basile, K. C., Gilbert, L. K., Merrick, M. T., Patel, N., Walling, M., & Jain, A. (2017). *The National Intimate Partner and Sexual Violence Survey (NISVS): 2010–2012 State Report.* National Center for Injury Prevention and Control, Centers for Disease Control and Prevention.

Smith Fawzi, M. C., Murphy, E., Pham, T., Lin, L., Poole, C., & Mollica, R. F. (1997). The validity of screening for post-traumatic stress disorder and major depression among Vietnamese political prisoners. *Acta Psychiatrica Scandinavica, 95,* 87–93.

Society for Personality Assessment. (n.d.). *Tele-Assessment of personality and psychopathology.* https://assets.noviams.com/novi-file-uploads/spa/PDFs___ Documents/COVID-19_Resources/Tele-Assessment_Resources/SPA_Personality_ Tele-Assessment-Guidance_6_10_20.pdf

Society for Personality Assessment. (2023). *COVID-19 resources: Tele-assessment resources.* https://www.personality.org/covid-19-resources

Somer, E., & Dell, P. F. (2005). Development of the Hebrew-Multidimensional Inventory of Dissociation (H-MID): A valid and reliable measure of pathological dissociation. *Journal of Trauma & Dissociation, 6*(1), 31–53. https://doi.org/10.1300/J229v06n01_03

Southwick, S. M., Krystal, J. H., Bremner, J. D., Morgan, C. A., III, Nicolaou, A. L., Nagy, L. M., Johnson, D. R., Heninger, G. R., & Charney, D. S. (1997). Noradrenergic and serotonergic function in posttraumatic stress disorder. *Archives of General Psychiatry, 54*(8), 749–758. https://doi.org/10.1001/archpsyc.1997.01830200083012

Spiegel, D., Koopman, C., Cardeña, E., & Classen, C. C. (1996). Dissociative symptoms in the diagnosis of acute stress disorder. In L. K. Michelson & W. J. Ray (Eds.), *Handbook of dissociation: Theoretical, empirical, and clinical perspectives* (pp. 367–380). Plenum Press.

Spiegel, D., Loewenstein, R. J., Lewis-Fernández, R., Sar, V., Simeon, D., Vermetten, E., Cardeña, E., & Dell, P. F. (2011). Dissociative disorders in DSM-5. *Depression and Anxiety, 28*(12), E17–E45. https://doi.org/10.1002/da.20923

Spinazzola, J., Hodgdon, H., Liang, L.-J., Ford, J. D., Layne, C. M., Pynoos, R., Briggs, E. C., Stolbach, B., & Kisiel, C. (2014). Unseen wounds: The contribution of psychological maltreatment to child and adolescent mental health and risk outcomes. *Psychological Trauma: Theory, Research, Practice, and Policy, 6*(Suppl. 1), S18–S28. https://doi.org/10.1037/a0037766

Spitzer, R. L. Williams, J. B., Gibbon, M., & First, M. B. (1990). *User's guide for the Structured Clinical Interview for DSM-III-R.* American Psychiatric Association.

Springs, F. E., & Friedrich, W. N. (1992). Health risk behaviors and medical sequelae of childhood sexual abuse. *Mayo Clinic Proceedings, 67*(6), 527–532. https://doi.org/10.1016/S0025-6196(12)60458-3

Sroufe, L. A., Egeland, B., Carlson, E., & Collins, W. A. (2005). Placing early attachment experiences in developmental context: The Minnesota Longitudinal Study. In K. E. Grossmann, K. Grossmann, & E. Waters (Eds.), *Attachment from infancy to adulthood: The major longitudinal studies* (pp. 48–70). Guilford Press.

Stadnik, R. D., Brand, B., & Savoca, A. (2013). Personality Assessment Inventory profile and predictors of elevations among dissociative disorder patients. *Journal of Trauma & Dissociation, 14*(5), 546–561. https://doi.org/10.1080/15299732.2013.792310

Stein, D. J., Grant, J. E., Franklin, M. E., Keuthen, N., Lochner, C., Singer, H. S., & Woods, D. W. (2010). Trichotillomania (hair pulling disorder), skin picking disorder, and stereotypic movement disorder: Toward DSM-V. *Depression and Anxiety, 27*(6), 611–626. https://doi.org/10.1002/da.20700

Steinberg, M. (1994). *Structured Clinical Interview for DSM-IV Dissociative Disorders– Revised (SCID-D-R)*. American Psychiatric Press.

Steinberg, M. (2023). *The SCID-D Interview: Dissociation assessment in therapy, forensics, and research*. American Psychiatric Association Publishing.

Stoltenborgh, M., van Ijzendoorn, M. H., Euser, E. M., & Bakermans-Kranenburg, M. J. (2011). A global perspective on child sexual abuse: Meta-analysis of prevalence around the world. *Child Maltreatment, 16*(2), 79–101. https:// doi.org/10.1177/1077559511403920

Strand, V. C., Sarmiento, T. L., & Pasquale, L. E. (2005). Assessment and screening tools for trauma in children and adolescents: A review. *Trauma, Violence & Abuse, 6*(1), 55–78. https://doi.org/10.1177/1524838004272559

Straus, M. A. (1979). Measuring intrafamily conflict and violence: The Conflicts Tactics (CT) Scales. *Journal of Marriage and Family, 41*(1), 75–88. https:// doi.org/10.2307/351733

Straus, M. A., Hamby, S. L., Finkelhor, D., Moore, D. W., & Runyan, D. (1998). Identification of child maltreatment with the Parent–Child Conflict Tactics Scales: Development and psychometric data for a national sample of American parents. *Child Abuse & Neglect, 22*(4), 249–270. https://doi.org/10.1016/ S0145-2134(97)00174-9

Sue, D. W., Capodilupo, C. M., Torino, G. C., Bucceri, J. M., Holder, A. M. B., Nadal, K. L., & Esquilin, M. (2007). Racial microaggressions in everyday life: Implications for clinical practice. *American Psychologist, 62*(4), 271–286. https://doi.org/10.1037/0003-066X.62.4.271

Sullivan, P. F. (2005). The genetics of schizophrenia. *PLoS Medicine, 2*(7), e212. https://doi.org/10.1371/journal.pmed.0020212

Tansill, E. C., Edwards, K. M., Kearns, M. C., Gidycz, C. A., & Calhoun, K. S. (2012). The mediating role of trauma-related symptoms in the relationship between sexual victimization and physical health symptomatology in undergraduate women. *Journal of Traumatic Stress, 25*(1), 79–85. https://doi.org/ 10.1002/jts.21666

Teicher, M. H., Gordon, J. B., & Nemeroff, C. B. (2022). Recognizing the importance of childhood maltreatment as a critical factor in psychiatric diagnoses, treatment, research, prevention, and education. *Molecular Psychiatry, 27*(3), 1331–1338. https://doi.org/10.1038/s41380-021-01367-9

Teicher, M. H., Samson, J. A., Polcari, A., & McGreenery, C. E. (2006). Sticks, stones, and hurtful words: Relative effects of various forms of childhood maltreatment. *American Journal of Psychiatry, 163*(6), 993–1000. https://doi.org/ 10.1176/ajp.2006.163.6.993

Thomas, K. M., Hopwood, C. J., Orlando, M. J., Weathers, F. W., & McDevitt-Murphy, M. E. (2012). Detecting feigned PTSD using the Personality Assessment Inventory. *Psychological Injury and Law, 5*(3), 192–201. https://doi.org/10.1007/s12207-011-9111-6

Thomas, N., Gurvich, C., & Kulkarni, J. (2019). Borderline personality disorder, trauma, and the hypothalamus–pituitary–adrenal axis. *Neuropsychiatric Disease and Treatment, 15,* 2601–2612. https://doi.org/10.2147/NDT.S198804

Tjaden, P., & Thoennes, N. (1998, November). *Prevalence, incidence, and consequences of violence against women: Findings from the National Violence Against Women Survey* [Research in brief]. U.S. Department of Justice, National Institute of Justice, and U.S. Department of Health and Human Services, Centers for Disease Control and Prevention. https://doi.org/10.1037/e330452004-001

Tjaden, P., & Thoennes, N. (2000, November). *Full report of the prevalence, incidence, and consequences of violence against women: Findings from the National Violence Against Women Survey* (NCJ Publication No. 183781). U.S. Department of Justice, Centers for Disease Control and Prevention. https://www.ojp.gov/pdffiles1/nij/183781.pdf

Ugarte, M., Zarate, L., & Farley, M. (2004). Prostitution and trafficking of women and children from Mexico to the United States. *Journal of Trauma Practice, 2*(3–4), 147–165. https://doi.org/10.1300/J189v02n03_08

Ullman, S. E., Relyea, M., Peter-Hagene, L., & Vasquez, A. L. (2013). Trauma histories, substance use coping, PTSD, and problem substance use among sexual assault victims. *Addictive Behaviors, 38*(6), 2219–2223. https://doi.org/10.1016/j.addbeh.2013.01.027

United Nations Treaty Collection. (1984). *Convention against torture and other cruel, inhuman or degrading treatment or punishment.* http://treaties.un.org/Pages/ViewDetails.aspx?srcTREATY&mtdsg_no=IV-9&chapter4&lang=en

Ursano, R. J., Fullerton, C. S., Epstein, R. S., Crowley, B., Vance, K., Kao, T. C., & Baum, A. (1999). Peritraumatic dissociation and posttraumatic stress disorder following motor vehicle accidents. *The American Journal of Psychiatry, 156*(11), 1808–1810. https://doi.org/10.1176/ajp.156.11.1808

U.S. Department of Health and Human Services. (2021). *Notification of enforcement discretion for telehealth remote communications during the COVID-19 nationwide public health emergency.* https://www.hhs.gov/hipaa/for-professionals/special-topics/emergency-preparedness/notification-enforcement-discretion-telehealth/index.html

U.S. Department of State. (2005). *Trafficking in persons report.* http://www.state.gov/j/tip/rls/tiprpt/2005

Vaillancourt-Morel, M.-P., Godbout, N., Labadie, C., Runtz, M., Lussier, Y., & Sabourin, S. (2015). Avoidant and compulsive sexual behaviors in male and female survivors of childhood sexual abuse. *Child Abuse & Neglect, 40,* 48–59. https://doi.org/10.1016/j.chiabu.2014.10.024

Vaishnavi, S., Payne, V., Connor, K., & Davidson, J. R. T. (2006). A comparison of the SPRINT and CAPS assessment scales for posttraumatic stress disorder. *Depression and Anxiety, 23*(7), 437–440. https://doi.org/10.1002/da.20202

Valera, R. J., Sawyer, R. G., & Schiraldi, G. R. (2000). Violence and post traumatic stress disorder in a sample of inner city street prostitutes. *American Journal of Health Studies, 16*, 149–155.

Van Bruggen, L. K., Runtz, M. G., & Kadlec, H. (2006). Sexual revictimization: The role of sexual self-esteem and dysfunctional sexual behaviors. *Child Maltreatment, 11*(2), 131–145. https://doi.org/10.1177/1077559505285780

Vance, M. C., Kovachy, B., Dong, M., & Bui, E. (2018). Peritraumatic distress: A review and synthesis of 15 years of research. *Journal of Clinical Psychology, 74*(9), 1457–1484. https://doi.org/10.1002/jclp.22612

van der Hart, O., van Dijke, A., van Son, M., & Steele, K. (2001). Somatoform dissociation in traumatized World War I combat soldiers: A neglected clinical heritage. *Journal of Trauma & Dissociation, 1*(4), 33–66. https://doi.org/10.1300/J229v01n04_03

van der Kolk, B. A. (2005). Developmental trauma disorder: Toward a rational diagnosis for children with complex trauma histories. *Psychiatric Annals, 35*(5), 401–408. https://doi.org/10.3928/00485713-20050501-06

van der Kolk, B. A., & Ducey, C. (1984). Clinical implications of the Rorschach in post-traumatic stress disorder. In B. A. van der Kolk (Ed.), *Post-traumatic stress disorder: Psychological and biological sequelae* (pp. 29–42). American Psychiatric Association.

van der Kolk, B. A., & Ducey, C. (1989). The psychological processing of traumatic experience: Rorschach patterns in PTSD. *Journal of Traumatic Stress, 2*(3), 259–274. https://doi.org/10.1002/jts.2490020303

van der Kolk, B. A., Roth, S., Pelcovitz, D., Sunday, S., & Spinazzola, J. (2005). Disorders of extreme stress: The empirical foundation of a complex adaptation to trauma. *Journal of Traumatic Stress, 18*(5), 389–399. https://doi.org/10.1002/jts.20047

van Dijke, A., Ford, J. D., van der Hart, O., van Son, M., van der Heijden, P., & Buhring, M. (2012). Complex posttraumatic stress disorder in patients with borderline personality disorder and somatoform disorders. *Psychological Trauma: Theory, Research, Practice, and Policy, 4*(2), 162–168. https://doi.org/10.1037/a0025732

van Ijzendoorn, M., & Schuengel, C. (1996). The measurement of dissociation in normal and clinical populations: Meta analytic validation of the Dissociative Experiences Scale (DES). *Clinical Psychology Review, 16*(5), 365–382. https://doi.org/10.1016/0272-7358(96)00006-2

Van Ommeren, M., de Jong, J. T. V. M., Sharma, B., Komproe, I., Thapa, S. B., & Cardeña, E. (2001). Psychiatric disorders among tortured Bhutanese refugees in Nepal. *Archives of General Psychiatry, 58*(5), 475–482. https://doi.org/10.1001/archpsyc.58.5.475

Vanwesenbeeck, I., de Graaf, R., van Zessen, G., Straver, C. J., & Visser, J. H. (1995). Professional HIV risk taking, levels of victimization, and well-being in female prostitutes in the Netherlands. *Archives of Sexual Behavior, 24*(5), 503–515. https://doi.org/10.1007/BF01541831

Viglione, D. J., Blume-Marcovici, A. C., Miller, H. L., Giromini, L., & Meyer, G. (2012). An inter-rater reliability study for the Rorschach performance assessment system. *Journal of Personality Assessment, 94*(6), 607–612. https://doi.org/ 10.1080/00223891.2012.684118

Viglione, D. J., de Ruiter, C., King, C. M., Meyer, G. J., Kivisto, A. J., Rubin, B. A., & Hunsley, J. (2022). Legal admissibility of the Rorschach and R-PAS: A review of research, practice, and case law. *Journal of Personality Assessment, 104*(2), 137-161. https://doi.org/10.1080/00223891.2022.2028795

Vigod, S. N., & Rochon, P. A. (2020). The impact of gender discrimination on a woman's mental health. *EClinicalMedicine, 20*, 100311. https://doi.org/ 10.1016/j.eclinm.2020.100311

Vogt, D., Smith, B. N., King, L. A., King, D. W., Knight, J., & Vasterling, J. J. (2013). Deployment Risk and Resilience Inventory-2 (DRRI-2): An updated tool for assessing psychosocial risk and resilience factors among service members and veterans. *Journal of Traumatic Stress, 26*(6), 710–717. https://doi.org/10.1002/jts.21868

Waller, N. G., Putnam, F. W., & Carlson, E. B. (1996). Types of dissociation and dissociative types: A taxometric analysis of dissociative experiences. *Psychological Methods, 1*(3), 300–321. https://doi.org/10.1037/1082-989X.1.3.300

Wang, Y., Chung, M. C., Wang, N., Yu, X., & Kenardy, J. (2021). Social support and posttraumatic stress disorder: A meta-analysis of longitudinal studies. *Clinical Psychology Review, 85*, 101998. https://doi.org/10.1016/j.cpr.2021.101998

Watson, C. G., Plemel, D., DeMotts, J., Howard, M. T., Tuorila, J., Moog, R., Thomas, D., & Anderson, D. (1994). A comparison of four PTSD measures' convergent validities in Vietnam veterans. *Journal of Traumatic Stress, 7*(1), 75–82. https://doi.org/10.1002/jts.2490070108

Weathers, F. W., Blake, D. D., Schnurr, P. P., Kaloupek, D. G., Marx, B. P., & Keane, T. M. (2013). *The Life Events Checklist for DSM-5 (LEC-5)*. https://www.ptsd. va.gov/professional/assessment/te-measures/life_events_checklist.asp

Weathers, F. W., Blake, D. D., Schnurr, P. P., Kaloupek, D. G., Marx, B. P., & Keane, T. M. (2013). *The Clinician-Administered PTSD Scale for DSM-5 (CAPS-5)*. https://www.ptsd.va.gov/professional/assessment/adult-int/caps.asp

Weathers, F. W., Bovin, M. J., Lee, D. J., Sloan, D. M., Schnurr, P. P., Kaloupek, D. G., Keane, T. M., & Marx, B. P. (2018). The Clinician-Administered PTSD Scale for *DSM-5* (CAPS-5): Development and initial psychometric evaluation in military veterans. *Psychological Assessment, 30*(3), 383–395. https://doi.org/ 10.1037/pas0000486

Weathers, F. W., Litz, B. T., Herman, D. S., Huska, J. A., & Keane, T. M. (1993, October). *The PTSD Checklist (PCL): Reliability, validity, and diagnostic utility* [Paper presentation]. Annual Convention of the International Society for Traumatic Stress Studies, San Antonio, TX, United States.

Weathers, F. W., Litz, B. T., Keane, T. M., Herman, D. S., Steinberg, H. R., Huska, J. A., & Kraemer, H. C. (1996). The utility of the SCL-90-R for the diagnosis of war-zone-related PTSD. *Journal of Traumatic Stress, 9*(1), 111–128.

Weathers, F. W., Litz, B. T., Keane, T. M., Palmieri, P. A., Marx, B. P., & Schnurr, P. P. (2013). The PTSD Checklist for *DSM-5* (PCL-5). https://www.ptsd.va.gov/professional/assessment/adult-sr/ptsd-checklist.asp

Webb, A., Heyne, G., Holmes, J. E., & Peta, J. L. (2016, April). Which box to check: Assessment norms for gender and the implications for transgender and nonbinary populations. *Division 44 Newsletter.* https://www.apadivisions.org/division-44/publications/newsletters/division/2016/04/nonbinary-populations

Weiner, I. B. (1996). Some observations on the validity of the Rorschach Inkblot Method. *Psychological Assessment, 8*(2), 206–213. https://doi.org/10.1037/1040-3590.8.2.206

Weiss, D. S., Brunet, A., Best, S. R., Metzler, T. J., Liberman, A., Pole, N., Fagan, J. A., & Marmar, C. R. (2010). Frequency and severity approaches to indexing exposure to trauma: The Critical Incident History Questionnaire for police officers. *Journal of Traumatic Stress, 23*(6), 734–743. https://doi.org/10.1002/jts.20576

Weiss, D. S., & Marmar, C. R. (1997). The Impact of Event Scale—Revised. In J. P. Wilson & T. Keane (Eds.), *Assessing psychological trauma and PTSD: A handbook for practitioners* (pp. 399–411). Guilford Press.

Weng, S. C., Chang, J. C., Yeh, M. K., Wang, S. M., Lee, C. S., & Chen, Y. H. (2018). Do stillbirth, miscarriage, and termination of pregnancy increase risks of attempted and completed suicide within a year? A population-based nested case-control study. *BJOG, 125*(8), 983–990. https://doi.org/10.1111/1471-0528.15105

West, C. M. (2002). Battered, black, and blue: An overview of violence in the lives of black women. *Women & Therapy, 25*(3–4), 5–27. https://doi.org/10.1300/J015v25n03_02

Wetter, M. W., Baer, R. A., Berry, D. T. R., Robison, L. H., & Sumpter, J. (1993). MMPI-2 profiles of motivated fakers given specific symptom information: A comparison to matched patients. *Psychological Assessment, 5*(3), 317–323. https://doi.org/10.1037/1040-3590.5.3.317

Wetzel, R. D., Murphy, G. E., Simons, A., Lustman, P., North, C., & Yutzy, S. (2003). What does the Keane PTSD scale of the MMPI measure? Repeated measurements in a group of patients with major depression. *Psychological Reports, 92*(3, Pt 1), 781–786. https://doi.org/10.2466/pr0.2003.92.3.781

Williams, L. M. (1994). Recall of childhood trauma: A prospective study of women's memories of child sexual abuse. *Journal of Consulting and Clinical Psychology, 62*(6), 1167–1176. https://doi.org/10.1037/0022-006X.62.6.1167

Williams, M. T. (2021). Racial microaggressions: Critical questions, state of the science, and new directions. *Perspectives on Psychological Science, 16*(5), 880–885. https://doi.org/10.1177/17456916211039209

Wilson, J. P., & Tang, C. S.-K. (Eds.). (2007). *Cross-cultural assessment of psychological trauma and PTSD.* Springer. https://doi.org/https://doi.org/10.1007/978-0-387-70990-1

Wilson, J. P., & Walker, A. J. (1990). Toward an MMPI trauma profile. *Journal of Traumatic Stress, 3*(1), 151–168. https://doi.org/10.1002/jts.2490030111

Wilson, L. C. (2018). The prevalence of military sexual trauma: A meta-analysis. *Trauma, Violence & Abuse, 19*(5), 584–597. https://doi.org/10.1177/1524838016683459

Wilson, R. S., Yung, A. R., & Morrison, A. P. (2020). Comorbidity rates of depression and anxiety in first episode psychosis: A systematic review and meta-analysis. *Schizophrenia Research, 216*, 322–329. https://doi.org/10.1016/j.schres.2019.11.035

Wolf, E. J., Mitchell, K. S., Sadeh, N., Hein, C., Fuhrman, I., Pietrzak, R. H., & Miller, M. W. (2017). The Dissociative Subtype of PTSD scale: Initial evaluation in a national sample of trauma-exposed veterans. *Assessment, 24*(4), 503–516. https://doi.org/10.1177/1073191115615212

Wolfe, D. A., Crooks, C. V., Lee, V., McIntyre-Smith, A., & Jaffe, P. G. (2003). The effects of children's exposure to domestic violence: A meta-analysis and critique. *Clinical Child and Family Psychology Review, 6*(3), 171–187. https://doi.org/10.1023/a:1024910416164

Wolfe, D. A., & McIsaac, C. (2011). Distinguishing between poor/dysfunctional parenting and child emotional maltreatment. *Child Abuse & Neglect, 35*(10), 802–813. https://doi.org/10.1016/j.chiabu.2010.12.009

Wolfe, J., Brown, P. J., & Bucsela, M. L. (1992). Symptom responses of female Vietnam veterans to Operation Desert Storm. *The American Journal of Psychiatry, 149*(5), 676–679.

Wood, J. M., Nezworski, M. T., Lilienfeld, S. O., & Garb, H. N. (2003). *What's wrong with the Rorschach? Science confronts the controversial inkblot test*. Jossey-Bass.

World Health Organization. (2000). *Women's mental health: An evidence based review.*

World Health Organization. (2022). *International Classification of Diseases and Related Health Problems* (11th rev.). https://icd.who.int/

Wright, D. B., & Loftus, E. F. (1999). Measuring dissociation: Comparison of alternative forms of the dissociative experiences scale. *The American Journal of Psychology, 112*(4), 497–519. https://doi.org/10.2307/1423648

Yamada, A.-M., & Marsella, A. J. (2013). The study of culture and psychopathology: Fundamental concepts and historic forces. In F. A. Paniagua & A.-M. Yamada (Eds.), *Handbook of multicultural mental health: Assessment and treatment of diverse populations* (2nd ed., pp. 3–23). Elsevier Academic Press. https://doi.org/10.1016/B978-0-12-394420-7.00001-1

Yates, T. M. (2004). The developmental psychopathology of self-injurious behavior: Compensatory regulation in posttraumatic adaptation. *Clinical Psychology Review, 24*(1), 35–74. https://doi.org/10.1016/j.cpr.2003.10.001

Yehuda, R., Kahana, B., Southwick, S. M., & Giller, E. L., Jr. (1994). Depressive features in Holocaust survivors with post-traumatic stress disorder. *Journal of Traumatic Stress, 7*(4), 699–704.

Young, A. M., Boyd, C., & Hubbell, A. (2000). Prostitution, drug use, and coping with psychological distress. *Journal of Drug Issues, 30*(4), 789–800. https://doi.org/10.1177/002204260003000407

Yun, J. Y., Shim, G., & Jeong, B. (2019). Verbal abuse related to self-esteem damage and unjust blame harms mental health and social interaction in college population. *Scientific Reports, 9*(1), 5655. https://doi.org/10.1038/s41598-019-42199-6

Zimmerman, M., & Mattia, J. I. (1999). Psychotic subtyping of major depressive disorder and posttraumatic stress disorder. *The Journal of Clinical Psychiatry, 60*(5), 311–314. https://doi.org/10.4088/JCP.v60n0508

Index

About the Authors

Erin M. Eadie, PhD, is a clinical and health psychologist in Toronto, Ontario, Canada. She is a staff psychologist for the South East Toronto Family Health Team and the head of child and adolescent care at the Fairmarc Psychology Centre. She conducts and publishes research on the impact of interpersonal trauma on mental and physical health, with a specific interest in posttraumatic stress, attachment, dissociation, and emotion dysregulation. Her clinical work and consultation focus on evidence-based assessment and treatment of trauma survivors across the lifespan.

John Briere, PhD, is professor emeritus of psychiatry and the behavioral sciences at the University of Southern California Keck School of Medicine. He is a past president of the International Society for Traumatic Stress Studies and is a recipient of the Award for Outstanding Contributions to the Science of Trauma Psychology from the American Psychological Association, the William N. Friedrich Lecturer: Outstanding Contribution to the Field of Child Psychology from the Mayo Clinic, and the Presidential Award for Contribution to Methods from the Association for Scientific Advancement in Psychological Injury and Law. He is author or coauthor of over 140 articles and chapters, 15 books, and 9 trauma-related psychological tests. His website address is (http://www.johnbriere.com/).